D0454771

Stronger, Faster, Smarter

Stronger, Faster, Smarter

A Guide to Your Most Powerful Body

RYAN FERGUSON

JEREMY P. TARCHER/PENGUIN
a member of Penguin Group (USA)
New York

JEREMY P. TARCHER/PENGUIN
Published by the Penguin Group
Penguin Group (USA) LLC
375 Hudson Street
New York, New York 10014

USA • Canada • UK • Ireland • Australia
New Zealand • India • South Africa • China

penguin.com
A Penguin Random House Company

Copyright © 2015 by Ryan Ferguson
Penguin supports copyright. Copyright fuels creativity, encourages diverse voices, promotes free speech,
and creates a vibrant culture. Thank you for buying an authorized edition of this book and for complying
with copyright laws by not reproducing, scanning, or distributing any part of it in any form without permission.
You are supporting writers and allowing Penguin to continue to publish books for every reader.

Most Tarcher/Penguin books are available at special quantity discounts for bulk purchase for sales
promotions, premiums, fund-raising, and educational needs. Special books or book excerpts also can be
created to fit specific needs. For details, write: Special.Markets@us.penguingroup.com.

Library of Congress Cataloging-in-Publication Data
Ferguson, Ryan.
Stronger, faster, smarter : a guide to your most powerful body / Ryan Ferguson.
p.   cm.
Includes index.
ISBN 978-0-399-17306-6
1. Physical fitness.   2. Exercise.   3. Muscle strength.   I. Title.
RA781.F457   2015   2014035246
613.7—dc23

Printed in the United States of America
1   3   5   7   9   10   8   6   4   2

BOOK DESIGN BY TANYA MAIBORODA

Neither the publisher nor the author is engaged in rendering professional advice or services to the individual
reader. The ideas, procedures, and suggestions contained in this book are not intended as a substitute
for consulting with your physician. All matters regarding your health require medical supervision.
Neither the author nor the publisher shall be liable or responsible for any loss or damage allegedly
arising from any information or suggestion in this book.

A Note of Gratitude

Many thanks are in order, for without the love, encouragement, support, and help I've received along the way, this book, my very first attempt at writing one, would almost certainly not exist.

I would like to first thank the two incredible individuals who played *the* central role of taking my crazy idea of a book from words handwritten on notebook paper in prison to something that felt real, professional, and, most important, presentable. If Myka Cain and James Dunn, a.k.a. Young Dizzle, hadn't believed in my drive and vision, this exercise in creativity would likely have been nothing more than a short-lived moment in time. Worse, I'd probably still be staring at notebooks full of chicken scratch and useful information with no clue of how to transfer it onto one of those things I hadn't seen in a decade . . . a computer! You two helped bring this to life with *a lot* of hard work, while not once asking for or expecting anything of me. Even more than for getting this book off the ground, I would like to thank both of you for showing me what true friendship is all about. As far as I am concerned, we are, and always will be, a team. I can't wait for the day you get out of there, James, so we can work, and work out, together once again. As you know, I'd acknowledge more of your editorial skills here, but I don't want the pettiness of prison to hamper your current existence.

Myka, my beautiful love, what can I even begin to say about you? So many times you have saved me on this book. The hours you've put in . . . you are an incredible woman! I don't know how you do it, but this should be your primary job. Editing, communications, design, technical skills, social media expert, you've got it all. And that's not even talking about your radiant personality and charming smile! I am one lucky man to have you in my life!

I'd also like to thank the individuals who helped on other aspects of this book, primarily reading it over for ways to improve it, as well as those who fought for my freedom and took the time to review the evidence, thus not only believing in my innocence but knowing of it. The reason for thanking both at once is because, more often than not, these people were one and the same. Richard Drew, your name pops up first in my mind, since you have been and continue to be a huge part of my life. I'm very lucky to have a friend who looks out for me as you have. Much love, man!

Ben Hamrah, Ashley Hennerich, Affton Hennerich, Mike Rognlien, Andrew Jenks, Anthony Galloway, Dylan Ratigan, Erin Moriarti, Gale Zimmerman, Jason Flom, and Chip Rosenbloom also come to mind here. I'm grateful for so many aspects of what you've done for me and this book. Whether you know it or not, you've all contributed a great deal to my success in not only various aspects of this book but also, and more important, my success in finding the freedom that had been unjustly taken from me.

Speaking of the fight for freedom, I must say a huge "thank-you" to the brilliant Doug Johnson and my "lifetime attorney," friend, adviser, and mentor, Kathleen Zellner. If not for their drive, passion, belief, and superior skill in the field of law, my family, my supporters, and I would likely still be fighting for justice.

Supporters! Yes, I have a special place in my heart for all of the beautiful people out there who have supported my family and me. It is you who showed me that even though there is much evil in the world, particularly from those in positions of authority, there is also an overwhelming abundance of kindness, generosity, and love. Just when I was about to give up on humanity, it is you who bonded to-gether, bringing me the gift of peace and happiness that comes with knowing you're part of something much larger: a worldwide family!

Which brings me to the last and ultimately most important people in this book, in the fight I've endured, and in my life in general: family. Bill Ferguson, Leslie Ferguson, Kelly Ferguson, Don and Kappy Frazier, Alberta Ferguson, Bob and Steve Frazier, the balance of the Fraziers, and the Norrises, as well as the rest of my extended family. Thank you so much to all of you for showing me what family is all about. I could not have made it through this past decade without you. This book wouldn't be a reality or have even been a dream of mine if you hadn't chosen to sacrifice, suffer, and endure the pain of the reality that held me hostage. You had the option not to care and I will never forget, or take that for granted. You are everything and I love you so much!

Especially Bill, Leslie, and Kelly Ferguson. No one in this world could have anticipated the brilliance of one family. Both in their fight and their love. I've said it a million times, but what's once more? I would be nothing without you. My life begins and ends with you three. Always. I love you.

Thank you.

—Ryan W. Ferguson

Contents

Preface

God asks no man whether he will accept life.
That is not the choice. You must take it. The only choice is how.

—HENRY WARD BEECHER

My Life Behind Bars

Hello, my name is Ryan Ferguson. Thank you for picking up my book. This is the story of a young man who came of age within the confines of a maximum-security prison. What makes this story unique is that this man was locked up for a crime he did not commit. In total, he lost nearly 10 years of his life. Friends turned their backs on him. The world called him a murderer and a liar. The experience could have broken him. Yet he chose to fight back and persevere. That man is me, and my story began on March 10, 2004. That was the date I was arrested for murder.

Over the last decade I have experienced more setbacks and defeats than most people experience in a whole lifetime. I have seen the inner workings of the U.S. justice system at its very worst and how the truth comes second to securing a conviction. I *never* gave up, though. I fought endlessly to prove my innocence, and now I continue to fight for others.

Once convicted, I was faced with two options: fight or flight. I was a terrified 19-year-old kid who had never been in trouble with the law and who suddenly found himself locked up in county jail and later in a maximum-security prison. It didn't seem possible. After the initial panic attacks subsided and I faced the grim reality of a possible life sentence staring down at me, the only thing I knew how to do was fight. Fight for my future; fight for my life; fight for my mind, my body; and, most important, my innocence. I knew I had to find a way. More than that, I had to find *my* way. My way to fight through the stresses, the pain, and the fear in order to make myself tougher.

Throughout this torturous journey I have endured many trials and tribulations that probably should have destroyed my strength, my hope, and even my will to carry on. That is not me, though. Backed by an incredible family and an overwhelming set of documented facts, I refused to allow someone to get away with taking my life for something they knew I did not do. As time went on, media attention rose and my case was featured on several national television news programs. Maybe you've seen these or know my story from another source. If not, I'll start with the basic facts. Here's where it all began: Halloween night 2001.

Around 2:10 a.m. on November 1, 2001, Kent Heitholt, sports editor for the *Columbia Daily Tribune*, logged off his computer and left his office in Columbia, Missouri. Within minutes he was savagely attacked and murdered next to his car in the newspaper's parking lot. A tragic death, Kent's murder shocked the local community.

Sitting in the empty lot that night was Kent Heitholt's colleague Michael Boyd. Boyd claimed the two spoke briefly and then he drove away at around 2:20 a.m. Heitholt, a large man standing six feet three and weighing 315 pounds, was struck from behind on his head multiple times and strangled with his own belt. Nothing of value was stolen from the victim, aside from possibly an inexpensive watch and his car keys.

The first people on the scene were two janitors, Shawna Ornt and Jerry Trump. Ornt had gone out for a break and observed two figures beside Heitholt's car. As suspicion mounted within her, she quickly retraced her steps and got her coworker Trump. The two peered out into the parking lot but couldn't see anything. Finally, Trump called out and two men stepped out from behind the car. The man at the rear of the car walked toward Ornt and spoke to her, saying, "Somebody's hurt, get help," before calmly rejoining the other man and walking away. Ornt got a good look at the man, including his face, before he left the scene. They then called 911 at 2:26 a.m.

Later that night, Shawna Ornt helped police create a composite drawing of the man who had spoken to her. Police considered her the "sole witness." Her colleague Jerry Trump was also questioned. Trump told the police, and later others, that he couldn't identify or give a detailed description of the individuals. Meanwhile, Boyd, the last known person to see Kent Heitholt alive, was only briefly questioned by the police and never investigated as a potential suspect.

Investigators discovered a trail of hair, blood, and fingerprints at the crime scene. The killer would likely have been covered in blood. There were also two sets of shoe prints leading away from the scene. A police K-9 unit tracked the scent from those shoe prints to a University of Missouri dorm. For the authorities there seemed to be a trove of evidence to follow, yet the murder of Kent Heitholt remained unsolved.

On the second anniversary of Heitholt's murder, the *Tribune* printed an article in hopes of gaining information about the unsolved murder. The article displayed the composite sketch that Shawna Ornt assisted investigators with and urged the community members to speak up if they had information about the murder.

For those in the Columbia Police Department who appeared so eager to crack the case that the facts became secondary, a lead arrived in the form of a troubled young man who read the newspaper article. Charles Erickson, a high school friend of mine, saw the composite sketch and thought it vaguely resembled him. He then appeared to have a dream that he was involved in the murder. On account of these newfound "images," Erickson began airing his fears and his dreams to his friends, including myself. Needless to say, I clearly remembered that Halloween night. Erickson and I had been at a local bar called By George. We left at closing time; I then drove him home and drove home myself. Erickson's dreams didn't make any sense. But his story was taken seriously by at least one friend, John Alder, who reported Erickson's dreams to the police. Following Alder's tip, for which there was a $10,000 reward, Erickson was picked up for questioning in March 2004.

What followed was one of the most shocking and disturbing police interrogations ever caught on camera. Erickson had no actual independent knowledge of the crime. He didn't know what the murder weapon was, how many times Kent Heitholt had been struck, or even where the murder had taken place. And those images from his dreams . . . not one of them fit the actual crime scene. Nevertheless, the police, desperate to clear up a high-profile cold case, proceeded to coerce and spoon-feed Erickson key unique details about the crime.

This, unfortunately, is where I came in. That morning, right outside of Kansas City, Missouri, was like any other. I was attending a history class at Maple Woods Community College and the only thing on my mind was the next day's exam. I had no worries. I had a decent job, good friends, an amazing family, and what I considered a bright future. All was going well until I left class and headed home. On the way there, two huge guys in an SUV were riding my bumper. This, of course, happens from time to time so I didn't think anything of it. Just a couple of douches with no respect. Nothing new. Once the lane I was in went from one to two, they stared me down as they passed. I soon turned off into my apartment parking lot, and no sooner had I put the car in park than that very same SUV flew up behind me, essentially blocking me in. My life would never be the same.

What followed was something I don't think I'll ever understand. These people I'd never seen before proceeded to treat me like the dirt on their shoes, rushing at me screaming "FBI," telling me not to move. From the arrest, to locking me in a car handcuffed with no explanation, to instantly and randomly stripping every right I had, things got intense. I didn't know what to make of it. I even thought for a time I was being arrested for a recent bomb threat at our school. I had no idea what was going on. I was totally and completely lost.

Within an hour I found myself in an interrogation room much like the ones you'd see in a bad movie. I told the police time and time again, over multiple hours of redundant questioning, that yes, I had been at the By George bar with Erickson on Halloween night 2001. I stated the obvious, that I had left around 1:30 a.m., when the bar closed. I told them repeatedly how I'd driven Erickson home before heading home myself. These were the simple facts and I never wavered from them.

In a neighboring room, however, while I sat there doing what I could to help, those same police were apparently doing what they could to wring a confession, right, wrong, or indifferent, from Erickson. Even though he had no personal knowledge of Heitholt's murder, and had stated multiple times that he'd blacked out and didn't know what happened after he left the bar, they didn't seem to care.

After many grueling hours of blatant threats and damning lies from the detectives, Erickson folded under the pressure. Assuming the police were being straight up with him about this false evidence, he figured he must have been present at the crime scene and simply told detectives what he thought they wanted to hear.

Over the following months, as Prosecutor Kevin Crane charged the two of us with murder, Erickson's statements slowly evolved, changing a number of times. Aided by "discovery," which contained fabricated police reports bolstering Erickson's supposed guilt and an exhaustive source of details about this crime, Erickson eventually came to believe his dreams were true; he and I had murdered Heitholt in a robbery gone wrong. Due to these false beliefs, and the fear that he must have committed the crime, Erickson panicked and agreed to a plea deal that would frame me for the murder of Heitholt in exchange for a lesser sentence for himself.

From the time of my arrest in March 2004 until my trial in October 2005, I found myself, a person convicted of no crime, trapped inside the county jail. Apparently those who wield the power within our criminal justice system find the Eighth Amendment of our Constitution to be nothing more than a joke. Case in point, the "Honorable" Judge Ellen Roper chose to ignore the whole "excessive bail shall not be required" part of the Constitution and gave me one for $20 million. The largest of its kind in history. We sought accountability for what appeared to be an outright senseless and slightly biased decision but found instead what would be the first of many indications that those within the justice system simply will not hold their colleagues responsible for their actions. Many wondered why I was even on trial in the first place, considering that Erickson's story was riddled with inconsistencies and flat-out impossibilities. None of the DNA evidence at the scene matched either Charles or me; there was absolutely no motive; I had no criminal background; and the ultimate reality was that there was, and would remain, zero evidence connecting me to this case.

But these same people had underestimated the indifference of the Columbia Police Department and an ambitious prosecutor, Kevin Crane. After multiple coaching sessions in Crane's office, the Charles Erickson who appeared before the jury was a new man. Confident and assured in his testimony, Erickson took the stand and pointed me out as responsible for the murder of Kent Heitholt. In so doing, he and Crane reenacted the supposed particulars of the murder, details Erickson had no knowledge of just a year earlier.

It was still far from an open-and-shut case. My attorneys fought back, barely. Partially because they didn't properly prepare for trial, a sad reality that plays out all too often once attorneys get your money, and partially because they weren't given all of the evidence to fight this case to begin with. This last issue of the defense not getting all of the information is actually illegal, but because our Supreme Court won't allow the law to hold police and prosecutors accountable for hiding evidence, it tends to happen in a vast majority of innocence cases. It's similar to making laws against drinking and driving where, instead of prosecuting those who are caught breaking this law with a felony and possible prison time, the courts would merely say, "Well, I'm sure you didn't mean to get drunk and run over those kids. How can you be responsible for them being on the road in the first place?" There is NO accountability. Just as drinking and driving would never stop if we didn't prosecute the offenders, police and prosecutors will continue to hide evidence and destroy countless lives if they know they won't even get so much as a slap on the wrist.

Nonetheless, Prosecutor Kevin Crane had a new "star witness" to place Erickson and me at the scene: janitor Jerry Trump. Though Trump had previously admitted he couldn't identify anyone at the scene, he now pointed me out in front of the jury as the man he had seen the night of the murder. Even more interesting was prosecutor Crane's choice *not* to ask Shawna Ornt, the police's "sole witness," if she could identify me as being there. Why ask Trump, who stated multiple times that he couldn't see the people in the parking lot, and not the sole witness, Ornt? Shawna Ornt later testified in a 2008 evidentiary hearing that she had met with Prosecutor Crane about three times prior to my trial. In that testimony, she said that she had told Crane numerous times that the men she saw that night were neither Erickson nor myself. Apparently, this information was not good enough for my attorneys or the jury to be made aware of.

After hearing just five days of evidence, which grimly coincided with my 21st birthday, the jury took the case into deliberation. Hours later they delivered their verdict. They found me guilty of first-degree robbery and second-degree murder. My sentence . . . 40 years behind bars. Happy 21st.

Instead of leaving 18 months of hard time in the county jail to the beauty of freedom, I'd instead be going to a place I never thought I'd see the inside of: state prison. I was shocked, betrayed, scared, lost . . . You name it and I was feeling it. It was a flood of the emotions you attempt to avoid in life. I could do nothing. I was powerless. I felt like the whole world was against me and the only people who could change that were the very ones who chose to defy the facts by choosing to put me in prison. I was left with so many questions. How could a jury convict me with no evidence? How long would it take to right this obvious wrong? How could those with the authority to serve and protect ignore the facts, and fight for what the documented evidence proved was so blatantly wrong? And the most pressing question, which may never be answered: How could they live with themselves?

This, thankfully, was not the end of my journey. Incensed by the jury's verdict and knowing I was innocent, my family made it their mission to uncover as much evidence as possible to prove my innocence. Devoting his life to the case, my father, Bill, eventually uncovered a shocking series of facts that would help prove that I should never have even been arrested, let alone tried or convicted.

Following my conviction in 2005, I was back in court several times over the years in a series of hopeless appeals. Each time the local judges ignored the facts of my case and, unsurprisingly, ruled against me. Unwilling to challenge the authority and judgments of their colleagues, none of these "ministers of justice" would be bold enough to stand in opposition to their peers. Sadly, as statistics show, this is typical for small-time judges. So, I sat in prison for years while these local hacks callously carried on with their country-club lives. This continued throughout many years of appeals, even though the only two witnesses against me would eventually take the stand, admitting to perjury. Remember, there was never any physical evidence linking me to Heitholt's murder and the "sole witness" to the crime scene had said I was not the person she saw in the parking lot. Could this really be how our justice system works?

Thankfully, back in October 2005, a few months before my trial, the media started to take an interest in my case. Over the years, three major news magazine shows ended up highlighting my family's extraordinary efforts, and their attention would prove invaluable in securing my eventual release. CBS's *48 Hours* and NBC's *Dateline* each ended up airing four episodes on the absurdity of this case. Later, ABC's *Nightline* also aired two detailed segments. I have since been interviewed by *Today*, *Good Morning America*, *The Early Show*, and *Katie*, Katie Couric's show. Beyond that were countless newspaper articles and posts written about my struggles and my family's. The world of fighting for yourself in the media is a story unto itself. It is a strange and difficult one for sure but ultimately gratifying once all the facts are exposed. All the media attention eventually attracted the interest of prominent defense attorney Kathleen Zellner. An extremely well-respected lawyer who focuses on appealing wrongful convictions, Kathleen and her brilliance and incredible work ethic were essential for the fight to come. In the fall of 2009, Zellner and her law partner, the unassumingly tenacious Doug Johnson, met with me and my family, examined the evidence, and realized there had been an obvious miscarriage of justice. They took my case pro bono, no expenses, and worked tirelessly to prove my innocence. Shortly after they came on board, an incredible break occurred in the case. Out of the blue I received some unexpected good news. In early November 2009, Charles Erickson had decided to come clean. In a handwritten statement, Erickson admitted he had lied under oath at trial!

Finally! After years of attempting to prove what was so obvious to a bunch of courts whose members wouldn't even listen to the evidence, the truth would reveal itself. I was still a bit frightened since I knew how these courts operated, but it felt like this hellish journey would soon come to its long-awaited conclusion. How could they *not* give me my life back when this man admitted to lying and all the evidence backed it up? For the first time in years I began to dream again. Later, things began to look even more promising. My defense team ended up speaking with the other witness, Jerry Trump, who confessed that he, too, had lied during his trial testimony under pressure from Prosecutor Kevin Crane. Apparently Crane had told Trump it would be "helpful to him" if Trump could place me at the scene of the crime, which clearly led to Trump's contrived story. Trump was fresh out of prison on an unrelated charge, and he was on parole when he was called into Kevin Crane's office. A classic scenario for the state to drum up false testimony. During his 2012 sworn habeas corpus testimony, Trump stated he was "scared out of his mind" during that unfortunate meeting and he was "under the guidance of the prosecutor's office."

When Erickson and Trump took the stand at my habeas corpus hearing in April 2012 and admitted they lied at my trial, both men subjected themselves to perjury charges. This had never happened before in an American courtroom during a habeas hearing. Recanting witnesses may give affidavits admitting perjury but they rarely take the stand under oath and admit perjury because this act can carry with it a potential 30-year prison sentence. Powerful! How else do you describe a moment like this in a case that was built on nothing more than words? What could possibly be more reliable than witnesses subjecting themselves to a veritable lifetime in prison just for coming clean?

This was it. My time had come, vindication had begun! It was a watershed moment in my case. Or so it seemed. Six months later, almost to the day of the 11th anniversary of Kent Heitholt's murder, Judge Daniel Green denied my appeal in the Cole County Circuit Court, stating that Trump's trial testimony had no weight in the jury's verdict and that Erickson's habeas testimony was "unreliable." What? Turns out Green had confused quite a few facts of my case, not to mention Missouri law. He didn't even understand the testimony in his own courtroom. A prime example is how he completely misstated a witness's, Kim Bennett's, testimony about where my car was parked at the By George nightclub in his 2012 finding. I was appalled. It felt as though he was intentionally attempting to alter the facts. What came out of the courtroom was so bad that I simply assumed he was completely out of touch with the facts he was ruling on. And that's being nice. How could a man given the responsibility to determine the course of another's entire future not even take the time to get the basic facts correct?

All those hopes and dreams about the future I thought I'd soon be having . . .

gone. Taken away in an instant. It looked like my future would be that of the only person in the United States to still be imprisoned with absolutely no evidence and with the only alleged eyewitnesses, whose testimony was key in my conviction, recanting in open court.

Nonetheless, we fought on. On January 31, 2013, my attorney filed a petition requesting a writ of habeas corpus from the Western District Court of Appeals, challenging Judge Daniel Green's ruling. At this time I was a bit wary and had little faith in Missouri courts. Even with no evidence and the only "witnesses" of this case recanting, Chris Koster, the Missouri attorney general, opposed the petition, calling it "a waste of judicial resources."

What could be worse than that? One no-name judge not doing his elected duty is bad enough, but the attorney general saying that he quite simply didn't care . . . heartbreaking. At that point, it really didn't feel as though anyone inside this privileged little bubble could have cared less about getting it right. Justice didn't exist. They essentially told us: "We'll never listen to your facts and arguments no matter how much proof you've got. You might as well get comfortable in your little cage."

At this point, I almost lost faith . . . almost. Even then I figured I'd give it one last shot. Oral arguments were just around the corner and this was pretty much the end of the line for me. If these people didn't feel it necessary to listen to the merit of our facts, no one else would. Chances were I'd spend the next 30 years listening to my celly snore as I attempted to sleep while a corrections officer shined a light in my eyes.

On September 10, 2013, my case was heard in front of the Western District Court of Appeals. I wasn't there but everyone I cared about was. It was a huge day. All the media even flew down. Looking back on that day I remember my girlfriend's phone dying just before the hearing started and a new friend of mine, film producer Andrew Jenks, giving her his so that we could finish our frantic conversation. Needless to say, it was a crazy time in my life.

Although the judges would not decide on anything during that hearing, I couldn't wait to hear how things went. After that phone call to my girlfriend, as everyone I knew went in and listened to my attorneys fight for my life, I had to go sit in my cell and hope to hear from someone soon how things transpired. All I could think was how surreal it was to have the center of my world so far away from me. I even wrote a post on Facebook about it, one of the many that would highlight my thoughts and feelings at the time. Don't get confused . . . I didn't have access to the Internet the entire time I was in prison. I recited a post to my girlfriend over the phone, so she could type it on her phone and then post it on Facebook. Anyway, later that day I received an ecstatic phone call from Kathleen saying that things went great. Better than even she could have hoped! I felt nothing. Maybe fear, sadness, or bewilderment but nothing like peace or joy. Even as I was able to speak to all those I loved and cared about, my emotions never changed. Everyone sounded great and felt more confident than ever, but for me it was just more of the same, I'd lost all faith. Hope no longer existed.

A couple of months went by, and on November 5, 2013, after I had spent nine years and eight months behind bars, the Western District Court of Appeals panel of judges ruled. It *finally* happened, they overturned my conviction! A week later, on November 12, 2013, they unexpectedly released me. I was a free man for the first time in nearly a decade! Chris Koster, the same attorney general who nine months earlier stated my case was a "waste of judicial resources," decided not to retry or pursue further legal action against me. Justice had finally won! I was

19 years old at the time of my arrest and released nearly 10 years later, less than a month after my 29th birthday. In total I spent nine years, eight months, and two days in prison for a murder I had no involvement in.

There are many blanks to fill in during those years, but that's for another book. What you've just read is the meat and potatoes of the life I was forced to endure. Every day I lost was a day I would never regain. While high school friends went off to college, graduated, pursued careers, married, and had children, I was behind bars. I missed the college experience, friends' weddings and the births of their children, celebrations, and even my grandmother's funeral. I eventually lost touch with many people whose lives had moved on while I remained falsely imprisoned. Life would never be the same.

My trials and conviction, however, are not what this book is about. The pages that follow are not about dry facts and the workings of the legal system. Instead this book is about my journey in prison and my experiences as one of the many wrongfully convicted men in America's justice system.

Prison is a severe form of mental torture. Through the days of this mental oppression and the physical hell of those first few years, I somehow managed to find a balance and was able to maintain most of my sanity. In this book, I highlight what I did to keep moving through the most oppressive time of my life, how I stayed focused, and what I learned along the way. I emerged from prison after almost 10 years not just unbroken *but* also stronger physically and mentally than I ever thought possible. This is the story of how I did it.

My hope is that this book will inspire you in your own life, too. It was initially written during my last five months of incarceration and much of it concerns my physical growth as I transformed myself from a skinny 19-year-old student into a wall of muscle. I had to in order to survive. Along the way, I'm going to explain, step-by-step, how I transformed my body, from exercises and routines to diet and daily habits.

But this isn't your typical fitness book. Sure, you'll pick up all the methods, tips, and ideas you need to get into the best shape of your life; but that ultimately is not what this book is all about. Many of you reading it will already be in good shape or may have no interest in packing on muscle. That's fine! I didn't set out to write a standard fitness book. I'm also *not* your typical fitness expert. I'm just giving you my personal experiences of how I transformed my body. If you want a typical fitness book, trust me, there are countless options on the shelves or online. *This*, though, *is better!*

Ultimately this book is about one word: GROWTH. If I can grow during what has been in many ways a truly terrible decade for me then so can you. Wherever you are, whoever you are, the only limits on you are the ones YOU impose on yourself. I was stuck in a concrete box for years and certainly had no advantages. This is the story of perseverance and determination, one celebrating our collective capacity to excel.

I *did not* give up hope, and I was not going to let the Missouri justice system define me. While in prison, I exercised my mind and body daily. I went to the physical extreme and fed my brain with knowledge. I wrote this book highlighting what got me through and gave me the sanity to continue my journey. For my last six years in prison, I even worked as a tutor three days a week helping other inmates study for their GED. Helping others helped keep me going.

My intention is for this to be the first of a series of books I plan on writing as I continue my personal journey. I will also highlight my efforts on my Facebook page (Freed Ryan Ferguson), which has over 100,000 (and counting) amazing supporters. Newer are my Twitter and Instagram accounts (@lifeafterten) and a website (www.RyanFergusonFitness.com). I now have a tremendous opportunity to reveal the ins and outs of our criminal justice system. I will use these platforms to help expose other cases of wrongful convictions, as well as to update people on my own life and personal growth.

Many people have wondered why I am writing this book now rather than simply telling the story of the last 10 years in a straight autobiography. The latter will share a story that will take time for me to tell properly, and there is also a great deal I must process in my own mind. My story is quite dense and complex; it's not one I want to rush. Don't worry, though, I'm working hard and it's coming. For your sake, for mine, and, most important, for all those who are currently wrongfully convicted, it has to be done right.

My point here is to prove that if I could make it in prison, where you're seen as nothing more than a number in a system that herds people like cattle through an inefficient, nonsensical bureaucracy, then you, too, can achieve great things no matter what life hands you. To the people who controlled my life for 10 years, I was little more than the dirt on their shoes, carelessly pushed around while they cashed a paycheck or scored a promotion. But that didn't stop me—and NOTHING in this world should ever stop you! Whatever we face, we can always find ways to become better.

I *know* my future is going to be amazing. I have been blessed with a once-in-a-lifetime opportunity, which I am committed to making the most of. I have a great support team: an incredible family, a wonderful girlfriend, fantastic friends, and countless allies in the legal and media worlds. I also know that I must take action in order to grow, and I want the same for you, too. So don't just read this book. USE IT!

There is no stopping you. The choice is yours. Take action. Take control of your life! Make every moment matter!

Introduction

*I know of no more encouraging fact than the unquestionable
ability of man to elevate his life by conscious endeavor.*

—HENRY DAVID THOREAU

Small Changes Equal Big Results

Many fitness books consist of nothing but pure, cold, hard facts. Dull, bland, and uninteresting. Others are stuffed full of life, emotion, and personal vicissitudes, thus taking the reader on a wild roller coaster ride while unfortunately lacking the information necessary for change. I cannot promise that what you are about to read will transcend these vehicles; however, the goal of this book is to marry these two concepts in order to inform, educate, and leave you in awe of what you're about to accomplish.

This book is, first and foremost, a tool. Its primary intention is to give the reader a clear and concise path to building the best possible physical version of him or herself without wasting time in the gym or the kitchen. Over and over again I've seen hoards of people attempt to get into shape only to end up quitting a few months or even a few weeks later. What has become obvious to me, after many years of observation, is that people are quitting not because of laziness, which is what I'd initially suspected, but because of the intense frustration of seeing lackluster results, which are the inevitable by-product of doing a lot of hard work *the wrong way*—in essence, wasting time spinning your wheels. Ernest Hemingway said it best when cautioning: "Never confuse motion with action." If used properly, the ideas contained in the next 10 chapters will eliminate all that useless movement and, thanks to the aid of education, will give your actions purpose.

The reason for 10 chapters is quite simple. Once I was able to untangle myself from all of the absurd, unrealistic expectations I'd built up in my mind thanks to many of the latest "two-minute fitness crazes," a clear path became increasingly evident. Ten necessary elements slowly began to reveal themselves as the core fundamentals to any health and fitness program. This pragmatic approach was an evolutionary leap forward for achieving not only the degree of physical success I'd experienced but also for the probability of my survival as an innocent man forced to live inside a maximum-security prison for what might be the remainder of my existence.

These steps encompassed the answers to nearly all of my goals: (1) get big so I can protect myself; (2) stay healthy so I don't get sick in a place where medical care is little more than two Tylenol and a pat on the back; and (3) safeguard my mind and my dreams against the overtly evil environment that I was forced to call home. My path was a perilous one and if I missed just one step, disaster was more than happy to greet me in the icy cold waters below.

Although our journeys will inevitably differ, we can all readily benefit from these simple concepts. It may seem a bit daunting at first, but I can assure you that through a few small changes taken from each chapter, you'll be well on your way to success. As far as I'm concerned, this isn't *a* path to success, this is *the* path to success. It's not always easy and it certainly isn't as simple as many charlatans might tell you, but *this is it*. This is what I wish I could have picked up and read 10 years ago. Nothing but the raw facts of what we need to do to look and feel good. The simple truth, presented in a concise manner, and made as attainable as possible from someone who has done it himself.

The simple reality is that by following the fundamental steps described in this book, you *can* have the body you want in the time you have. That said, in order to do this you must evolve your thinking and understand that it's all about working smarter, not harder! The whole idea is that through attaining knowledge and understanding the "whats, whens, and hows" of your diet and exercise habits, you'll be able to accomplish *more in less time*. As far as I'm concerned it's just that easy.

We will be able to achieve this by focusing primarily on the three main components that comprise this outlook: your workout; your diet; and your continued education, which will transform your daily activities. These components have been broken down and designed in such a way that each individual can immediately begin implementing changes, both large and small, into his or her lifestyle at his or her own pace, without too much disruption of normal activities. From here, we will be able to see and feel positive changes over time, which will inevitably aid and motivate us to make even more changes as we become comfortable with our progress and are increasingly encouraged by our results.

The basic reality that we all must face is that change takes time and that that is okay. The sooner we accept this, the sooner we'll see what we want looking back at us from the mirror. All that's needed is to start making whatever changes you feel comfortable with, and try adding something new each week. Remember, the more changes you make the better your results WILL BE.

Small Changes, Big Results

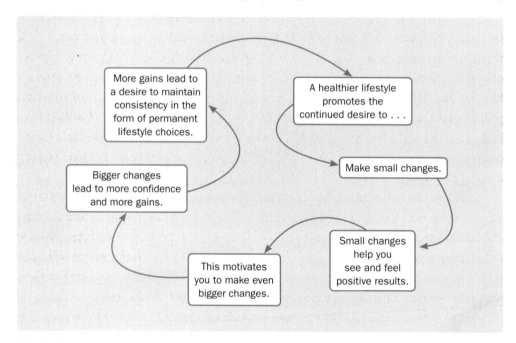

Who Can Benefit from This Lifestyle?

For a while now, I have struggled with how to describe this book's target audience. Who will this book be helping most? What is the central theme? Who can it most help? That's when I realized it shouldn't have to be so specific. Why should a book composed of research ranging from living longer to bodybuilding science and women's health to sports science be focused primarily on one group of people? This dynamic approach includes everyone!

Although it was initially intended for guys like myself who wanted that muscular, athletic beach body, but were tired of reading endless books and magazines that contradicted one another, it turned into an all-inclusive guidebook that presents the necessary information for attaining phenomenal health in one accessible volume. Much like my own goals and desires, the primary goal of this text progressed to a point where mental and physical health were just as important as body aesthetics. These are things I believe we all want, need, and desire to some degree—especially if they can be achieved through a series of smaller, readily achievable lifestyle changes.

Throughout my decade-long evolution, it became clear to me that when attempting to create our best physical selves, the same basic principles of workout, diet, and mentality apply across genders and lifestyles. Whether young or aging, skinny or big-boned, male or female, if we choose the right diet, at the right time, with the right workout for a sustained period of time, we can all attain the body we want with less work and be not only healthier but also happier for a lifetime.

In my opinion, as a typical person just trying to get into better shape and look good, this book encompasses what I believe other fitness books and magazines *should* be telling you but most often do not. Instead, they put us on overload with the minutiae in hopes of getting us to come back time and time again to buy more worthless or partially useful products. Although I go into great detail about my story, and the evolutionary process I went through, it's not really about my story. It's about you. It's about you and your story. It's about you accomplishing your goals and seeing the body and the life you want.

This book is essentially a guide to show you that even under the most extreme circumstances, YOU have the power to transform into the best-possible version of yourself. My story is merely here as an example to show you why I am so incredibly passionate about each and every word you will soon read. To show you that if *I* can do it, YOU can too! Thus illuminating how an extraordinarily *ordinary* person such as myself can transform his body, mind, and spirit using these basic, well-established principles.

We all have our own stories, our own personal struggles, which we must contend with daily. My personal story may seem extreme, but, in reality, these events and circumstances are only as powerful as we perceive and allow them to be. Who's to say my story is more life-altering than yours? No one. All you can do is pick yourself up and choose to be a survivor! Choose to give the time and dedication to do for yourself what no one else will. Choose to engage in creating the best life possible for yourself. This is simply the story of how I personally did it, which is why I believe we can ALL benefit from these life-enhancing habits.

How Vanity Makes Us Better

Let's be realistic. How many of us go out and buy books on fitness and exercise because our sole desire is to be "healthier"? If your answer was anything other than a laugh, then you're a better person than me. All I know is that I want to look good, period. At least that's how I started out. Although some may say this is superficial and the wrong reason for getting into shape (and they may very well be right), the fact remains that it's the number one reason people pick up this kind of book.

Some of you will read this book because of my story, of which there is a whole lot just for you, but if not, stop and think for a moment about *why* you bought this book. If you're being honest with yourself, the likelihood is that your desires are in line not only with mine but with millions of others who want to look good. Who *doesn't* want to look their best? Quite simply, it just makes life easier. You have more confidence, more energy, more pizzazz, and, whether right or wrong, people are more likely to gravitate toward you. Studies have also shown that finding jobs or enjoying benefits such as upward mobility are more readily accessible as well. And who knew about the laundry list of positive aspects as they pertain to your sex life? Google it! (I wouldn't know personally, as I've missed out on the past decade of life, but that is what "they" say.)

There's one other incredible benefit I want to touch on briefly, one that we'll address in depth later, and it's about how you start gaining the residual effects of actually feeling better mentally. At this point, health, short-term and long-term, tends to take hold, and you'll likely become a full-blown "health nut." It may take some time to reach this point, but mark my words, if you stick with it long enough, IT WILL HAPPEN! Ask any person you see with an above-average physique, or any friends and coworkers who have transformed themselves, and nine times out of 10 they will tell you how their desires went from pure aesthetics to overall health. Aesthetics, of course, remain a predominant factor.

My point is this: regardless of why you begin this quest, the reality is that you're making a better you. As you begin to feel great and see gains, that better you, in turn, will want to keep getting better and better. So, as far as I'm concerned, any reason—shallow or not—is a good reason to get started. Just venture down this path and you'll reach your destination soon enough. But I must note that, while this process contains relatively few steps, it certainly isn't child's play, and it requires a great deal of determination, effort, and energy. The harder you work and the more disciplined you are, the sooner you will begin to see the fruits of your labor.

Before We Begin

At this point, before we reach the good stuff, I'd like to make it clear that I am no "expert" on these subjects. The list of things *I am not* is far greater than the list of things that I am. The former list is quite extensive and includes such things as a personal trainer, nutritionist, physical therapist, or even an author. I mention this for two reasons. First, my goal is to improve your life, much in the same way that this program has improved mine. That said, you should always consult with your doctor before undertaking any physical, mental, or nutritional regimen. This book contains all of the key components necessary for you to change your body. A portion of the information I've chosen to share in this book has come from various sources such as university studies and research by doctors, nutritionists, sleep experts, and so on. This is my sincerest attempt at a safe and simple starting point, but, as you will often hear throughout the book, you must find what works best for you. ALWAYS PRACTICE CAUTION!

The second reason that I mention my lack of qualifications is because I believe this is precisely what makes the book so special. What do experts in physical therapy, nutrition, sleep, and working out have in common? They all know a lot about *one* particular subject. They are also absolutely necessary in their chosen fields and offer far more expertise than I could ever hope to share. But how many of them can competently combine all these subjects in a practically applicable way? How many have the real-world experience of experimenting with their own bodies for nearly a decade in the harshest of environments? How many have the perspective of a layperson, someone like you and me, who's fed up with all the confusing nonsense out there pulling you in a multitude of directions? None that I've ever come across, that's for sure.

I, however, have the experience. I've been pulled in all those directions. I've tried them all. At this point, I've sacrificed my poor mind and body during more than a decade of trial and error—something most experts have never done—and that's why I believe this book is so special. We could get caught up in all the small details to which the single-field experts must generally adhere; however, the majority of that information is not necessary to begin attaining the body of your dreams.

Consider this your foundation, if you will. The acquisition of a strong, competent base, which has been laid out in the following pages, will not only get you moving along the path toward realizing your dreams, it will also provide the support necessary for sustainable growth. Continue down this realistic road less traveled and you WILL be amazed before you are halfway through.

For the record, that was an opinion you just read: one that I believe in 100 percent, largely due to having experienced firsthand everything you are about to read. Many other opinions about such things as workouts, ease and simplicity of certain endeavors, and fitness or prison in general are discussed as well. All that can be said is that I call it how I see it and say what I believe in, so feel free to take what you read with a grain of salt if you like. I always do.

A New Dawn

Fortunately for you this is what you need to know to get you where you want to be, from a guy who has read it all, extracted all the necessary information from hundreds of books and magazines, cut out the fat, and, most important, has tried it all on himself. This is it. This is what you've been waiting for! There's also a decent story about my journey through prison as an innocent man looking to stay safe while attempting to perfect his body the easy way.

The conclusion: DON'T WASTE TIME, GET EDUCATED! For years now, people have commented on my work ethic. When I'm in the gym, I go *hard*. I push myself to the limits in order to get the most out of whatever time I'm willing to spend toiling away under the weights or on the track. When people ask how I'm able to push myself so hard and maintain consistency in my health regimen, my answer is simple: *I'm actually lazy.*

On the outside, and if looked at from our current perspective, this may seem like a joke, farcical in so far as it contradicts the solid work ethic that drew people to me in the first place. But this truth is, to me, just a simple fact. From what I've observed, most people, myself included, want to be in shape. Who says, "I'd like to be considered morbidly obese" or "Man, I wish I had a few more pounds around my hips"? NO ONE. The problem is that many of us, as we progress through the seasons of life, hit droughts. Droughts where our physical activity has dropped off. Droughts in our diets, when parties and holidays take over and we realize that, in the blink of an eye, we've been consuming terrible food for a month, three months, or a year. Even droughts where we simply choose to no longer care about our health or our bodies at all. Who among us can say that they've never lost for a time their motivation, their will, and their desire to be better?

We must be wary of these droughts, however, because when they hit us, they consume far more than just the present. These quiet, unassuming assassins consume our future—and it's not just the immediate future I'm concerned about. We can end up spending inordinate amounts of time and money on ridiculous diets trying to get back on track, compromising our long-term future. Lack of exercise, terrible diets, and the accumulation of fat and its by-products poisoning our systems over time will steal years from our lives. What's worse and thought of less often is that the quality of life in our remaining years will be plagued with disease, unnecessary suffering, and a revolving door of hospital visits. Who wants that?

Managing multiple chronic illnesses, the unnecessary strain of built-up stress, and the never-ending quest of trying to get back in shape . . . sound good to you? To me, all of this seems like a lot more hard work than investing a little of the now in positive lifestyle choices. If you take the simple steps laid out in this book, you can largely avoid much of this unnecessary suffering. Through putting in at least a minimal effort to *consistently* eat right, exercise, and maintain your health, your workload will be significantly less taxing and, more important, easier on your body.

So yes, I'm 100 percent serious when I say I'm lazy. Getting back into shape is far more difficult than staying in shape will ever be. So by staying in shape, I'm saving myself loads of time, money, and dignity. And this doesn't even get into the fact that the quality of life spoken of earlier will almost certainly be at a sustainably higher level. When considering our health, we must be *forward thinkers*. What we do now (eat, drink, exercise) determines our future. Think of your time and habits as an investment. Pay in a little each day, remain aware, and stay educated about your investments and then coast off into the sunset enjoying life as you age. Ignore these realities and the future is no longer in your control. Although a joke, I've always liked what comedian Redd Foxx had to say about us lovers of health: "Health nuts are going to feel stupid someday, lying in hospitals dying of nothing." Ha, well Redd, that's a good one—but at least I'll have gotten the absolute most out of life. Whether it be one day more, ten years more, or just better quality in the years I've got, the opportunity to be here on spaceship mother earth, kicking back and enjoying the ride, is all worth it.

So here is your all-inclusive guide: all you need to know, in one place, at one time, to get yourself started down the path to a better you. What's more is that I know how difficult this journey can be, since it is one I have been living for the past decade of my life. We all have our own time constraints and difficulties, but I assure you, if I can do it under the circumstances you'll read about in this book, YOU CAN TOO! *So start being lazy now by implementing these changes* and you'll soon be leaping into your new life. You'll thank me when you're lying on the beach in your sunset years, with your six-pack (abs that is), drinking a six-pack (of beer, of course), following a good game of tennis with your grandkids, and enjoying your life. Best of luck, my friends!

A Note to Women

The myth that women shouldn't lift weights is only
perpetuated by women who fear strength and men who fear women.

—UNKNOWN

Why a Note for the Ladies?

Although the principles for a healthy, well-balanced lifestyle outlined in this book are for everyone, of nearly any age, both men and women, I thought it important to take a moment (further urged on by my girlfriend, who is also an avid believer in the benefits of this healthy lifestyle) to speak directly to women readers. Ideally these few short pages will clear up some of the most common misconceptions around women's fitness, so that we can all move forward together into the bodies we want and deserve.

Due to all the fads, pseudodiets, and infomercials trying to sell the latest rinky-dink machine or butt-lifting workout, you ladies have been fed a lot of useless and counterproductive information. We all have, but society plays a big role in confusing the average woman even moreso, mostly because the media, for reasons I have yet to understand, seems to push the supermodel body on you from the womb to the tomb. It makes no sense because almost NONE of the guys I have ever known find this look to be exceptionally flattering. (That is, of course, in reality at least. If, however, you plan on living your life in print, the supermodel look may work for you.) For the most part, we males respect and desire a healthy, happy woman who eats a well-balanced diet (not just low carbs) and who has a little shape to her. Essentially what is generally considered most attractive is often most natural. Stick figures, in comparison, are not natural. But who cares what guys want? What's important is what *you* want and what matters to *you*. That being said, it must be noted, once more, that this lifestyle, workout included, *is for you, too*. Although everyone has different body types (guys are different from other guys, while girls are different from other girls), the reality is that guys and girls are physiologically very much the same in terms of how we gain and lose both fat and muscle. So let's take a look at how these fundamental similarities operate.

Should Women Lift Weights?

The single most important difference in fitness between the two sexes is that women develop muscle mass at a much slower rate than men—that's it, which is why I believe this workout is universal and designed for everyone. Because this workout incorporates foundational movements, it delivers the most desired and sought-after body type for *both* men and women, even though the end goal (lean muscle mass) is slightly different from a visual perspective. As men gain the muscle necessary to give them a masculine, athletic body type, women also gain the toned athletic look but without the mass. Multiple studies also suggest that weight training has an even more important place in women's lives; it can aid in bone densification, which helps solve a prevalent concern for aging women about bone-density loss. Otherwise, the two sexes are very similar in terms of the need for weight training and the vast array of health-related benefits they accrue from it.

How is this possible, you may ask? The science is complicated but the predominant differentiating factor is testosterone. This hormone, which men have in far larger quantities than women, helps men grow larger while women will generally stay smaller and get leaner due to their body not producing high levels of the substance. My point is that YOU WILL NOT GET TOO BIG! I often hear women say that they avoid weights because they don't want to gain mass and look all "manly." Sound familiar? I get it, though. While some may want this look, this book is for those of us in the middle who just want to look naturally healthy, lean, and athletic.

The reality is that it is extremely difficult to gain mass. The volume of work necessary for a man to do so is quite intense and grueling; and, given the physiological differences, for a woman to do so requires more or less doubling a man's efforts. This is why I can promise that you will not gain unsightly mass or have manly muscles. Even if you did, that wouldn't be a bad thing because that means you've met and surpassed your goals. It's a lot easier to lose muscle than it is to gain (trust me), so if this were the case, all you would have to do is stop.

Think about it: If gaining mass were so easy, wouldn't all your guy friends go to the gym every now and then and come out looking like Ryan Gosling or Mark Wahlberg? The reason they don't is because it takes a lot of very specific training, a very particular diet, and copious amounts of hard work. In order to get there, it would have to be a very deliberate goal on which you focused all of your energies. You'd have to lift heavy, work out more than most lifestyles would allow, and consume massive quantities of food to feed those Herculean muscles. If you want to get that big, good luck. It ain't easy and you'll have to find another book. While desirable for some, this quite simply is not our goal.

On the off chance that you do start gaining a little unwanted muscle, there is one simple solution. As we said earlier, just stop working out. If you ever begin to feel like you're getting too much out of your workout (although this is quite rare), all you have to do is take some time off and all that hard work will slowly begin to vanish.

This also brings up one of the most unfortunate things about exercise and fitness, which seems to continuously boggle my mind. You've got to stay on top of it . . . FOREVER. Once you get your body exactly how you desire it to be, you CANNOT STOP. If you do . . . poof . . . it'll vanish into thin air. We are all created equal in terms of losing gains from hard work, so unfortunately, this goes for everyone. Welcome to the importance of consistency.

It has also been brought to my attention that these days there is a large emphasis on women attempting to perfect their backsides. There are many ways to work on this muscle (that's what it is), but one remains king no matter how people attempt to view it. The squat. This is, was, and always will be your butt's best friend. The simple reality is the harder and heavier you go, the more you'll have to hold and to love until death do you part. There are many other supplemental workouts for your glutes, such as glute ham raises or bridges, but by forgoing this primary move, as both men and women often sadly do, you'll likely never see Beyoncé-esque images staring back at you from your full-length mirror. Add the stair stepper to this mix and you'll be well on your way to legs fit for the silver screen: toned, shapely, and seductive. What more could you want? That's why I love the stair-stepper contraption as a supplement to my squats. It gives me that extra burn in the legs, and it's a way of doing cardio while still building better hams, thighs, and, of course, those all-important glutes! I only mention the stair stepper here because I know that many women will actually use it, whereas guys often will not. If you think your friends can be finicky, then you've never seen a bunch of guys in the gym. The way they run from those stair steppers would make you think it was a yogurt-dispensing Shake Weight. Pathetic!

Come to think of it, I may need a guys' chapter, too. While women shouldn't be wary of protein powders and weights, men shouldn't be afraid of stair steppers, yoga, and Pilates. It's all relevant and useful to *everyone*! Heck, I do it all and my ego seems to be intact. No problems here; it's all about education. With this knowledge, I continue to diversify what I do, while managing to look and feel better than ever. Even if some may disagree, I know, thanks to understanding why some things are good for me and others aren't, that I'm physically healthier and physiologically better off than ever. We just have to get over ourselves. So as you can see, the notion that lifting weights is for men only is pure garbage. DON'T BUY INTO IT.

The Art of Counting Calories

This leads me to one of the most common misunderstandings that derails women's physical progress. Apparently, ladies (more so than men, who seem to get a thrill out of shoving food in their mouths in a rather Neanderthal fashion) tend to feel comfortable eating anything so long as they do it "responsibly." And many generally eat "responsibly" by keeping their caloric intake at an alarmingly low level. This misunderstanding of the need to count calories can quickly become an inhibitor of progress if acted on. It's important to note that counting calories is more a matter of science than just another numbers game. Although men, too, subscribe to this method of madness, albeit in significantly lower numbers, I cannot stress how detrimental this is to your overall health and progress in the gym.

First of all, you must take into account the nutritional differences of the types of food you eat. Although you may be consuming fewer calories, it may take far more work to burn these off than if you consumed 20 to 30 percent more calories from food of a different variety. If done correctly, you could consume more food, feel full for a longer period of time, and burn what you consumed at a faster rate than if you consumed fewer calories of a less nutritional profile. This brings up the second and most important aspect of food, which is the nutritional quality of the calories you consume. If, for instance, you take in 300 calories of food with a poor nutritional profile, such as a plain white bagel with cream cheese, you'd be getting almost zero nutrients or proteins and loads of simple, bad carbs and fats. If you instead ate 300 calories of food with a healthy nutritional profile, such as steel-cut oatmeal with peanut butter and bananas, you'd be getting vitamins A, C, and D; complex, good carbs; and a quality source of protein. Plus, you'll likely burn it all off faster due to how our bodies would use these nutrients.

For example, one day I ate an 800-calorie Blimpie sandwich in the prison visiting room. Eight hundred calories is quite a significant meal, so you think that would fill me up, right? It didn't. There wasn't even a whole lot to it, since it contained a little meat and cheese, white bread, and some dressing. Because the sandwich had no complex carbs, very little protein, and virtually no other nutrients, not only did I *not* get full, it had almost zero health benefits, which just made things worse. In contrast, the day after, I made myself a bowl of fresh vegetables with four ounces of chicken, ate a piece of wheat bread, and had a protein bar.

This left me stuffed and as an added bonus I got all kinds of proteins, complex carbs, and other essential nutrients. The best part was . . . this meal was only 600 calories. One small meal change, one *huge* difference.

Does Protein Make Women Fat?

While on the subject of calories, I'd like to debunk a long-held myth among women about protein supplements. PROTEIN SUPPLEMENTS WON'T MAKE YOU FAT! I swear this comes from the movie *Mean Girls* but then again, I suppose this myth has likely been around longer than the movie itself.

In short, as we'll touch on in depth in Chapter 6, protein, taken in adequate amounts, pre- and postworkout, will only give you better gains and faster results, while also promoting a more efficient recovery process. This is because muscle is made primarily of protein and water, so when you break down whatever amount of muscle you've currently got by working out, all this additional protein will help feed your muscle recovery with nourishment for lean growth. For maximum gains, studies recommend aiming to consume at least 20 grams of whey protein post-workout. Recent studies also show that consuming casein along with whey protein will further increase your results postworkout. Although protein is absorbed at very different rates (whey fast and casein slow with egg, beef, hemp, and other protein sources falling somewhere in between) depending on a plethora of factors, I would still aim to consume between 20 to 40 grams from one source or another every two to three hours. Ideally from a natural source but powders and bars are great alternatives that are used by some of the world's healthiest men and women. Remember, though, total daily consumption is by far more important than all the conflicting data of how often to eat this particular macronutrient. If you stick to this number, all of these "extra" calories will be absorbed for good use and will NOT be left to turn into fat.

What Can We Take from This?

So go out and eat, eat a lot, don't be afraid of protein, and don't be afraid to work out with weights. Work out with the guys even. I know it may feel out of place, but that's where you belong. We respect that! Show us what you're made of. Go hard, see what your body will do, and see what works for you. The weights will get you lean and toned in ways that aerobic exercising, plyometrics, and yoga never will. Remember, though, we're all different, so what works for you may not work for your bestie.

None of this is to say you should discontinue what some thoughtlessly and in my opinion wrongly refer to as "feminine" workout staples. They have an important place in fitness for everyone, including myself. Remember, it's all about balance. Throughout the week I do all types of these workouts: those that address the all-important hip abductors and adductors; yoga; and, of course, the stair stepper. These "girly" workouts are kind of like supplements to me. Added value, not replacements, to the fundamentals of the Big Six, which you'll read about later.

Now go eat and push some weights!

The Body

||||||||||||||||||||||||||||||||||||||||||||||||||||||||||||||||||||||||||||||||||||||||||||||||||||||||||||||||||||||||||||||||||||||||||||||

We should conduct ourselves not as if we ought to
live for the body, but as if we could not live without it.

—SENECA THE YOUNGER

1

Do what you can, with what you have, where you are.

—THEODORE ROOSEVELT

Fight or Flight

As a 19-year-old man in prison for a crime I didn't commit, I faced a very simple choice, a choice I can boil down into three very simple words. FIGHT OR FLIGHT.

The fact is, I could either try to run and hide from the potential horrors that faced me in prison, an option that even if successful would likely have left me in complete isolation for the rest of my life (they put these "subhuman wimps" in solitary confinement). Or, I could choose to SURVIVE. To face my fears. To stand up tall, back to the wall, and fight for myself. I chose the latter. And honestly, it's one of the reasons I'm here today, writing this as a free man.

My situation was extreme, of course. But we all, to different degrees, reach a point where we must face a similarly daunting choice in our lives. The question is: *What would you choose?* Do you stand up to your bullying boss or retreat to your "safe" cubicle and keep your head down? Do you allow your significant other to belittle you or do you fight for an equal relationship? Are you a people pleaser or have you learned to put your foot down and just be yourself?

What about your own body? Do you fight for your health or have you given up and essentially taken "flight"? How many of you continually put off your diet for another day, another week, another New Year, a "promised" day that never comes? Do you continually vow to join that gym and then feed yourself an endless diet of excuses: "I don't have the money," "I'm too tired," "I don't have time." At what point are you going to decide ENOUGH IS ENOUGH, it's time to fight back???

That's the decision I had to make, only the stakes weren't domestic or job related. They were life or death. As you can imagine, it was scary, difficult, and stressful, but this was *my* choice! One of the very few I had left. Making that choice made me feel alive. It made me aware that I was still a person. part of the human race . . . something and someone who demanded at least a bit of respect. A SHRED OF DIGNITY!

Early on in my incarceration I decided I was going to stand my ground. I was going to fight! Not only for my sanity and survival, but also against anything or anyone aiming to cause me harm. Obviously I wasn't looking for a fight. As a five foot nine, 160-pound man who had barely thrown a punch in his life, any tussle likely wouldn't end in my favor. Put it this way, I wasn't exactly serving time with men who had never used their fists before. What's more, many of these guys, several of whom would likely never live as free men again, had little to lose. I, however, wanted to walk out of prison still maintaining all my major bodily functions.

It is difficult to translate my thoughts at that time into words. I was faced with the decision to either check in (be locked up all day in protective custody), or go to the yard (join the mass of convicts and take whatever was coming my way). Actually, come to think of it, it's pretty easy to express how I felt. I was SCARED AS HELL!

Walking through that jail, all I could think was: "Don't show them you're scared, be yourself, and, if necessary, take an ass whooping or two to let them know you're more trouble than it's worth." I figured that wounds would heal and bruises would go away, but once you tuck your tail and run, the scars from permanent isolation would never subside. If I took flight I would never be free. So, with the mentality of "how bad can an ass whoopin' be?" I went in and got my respect. That is until I got my ass whooped!

I'll never forget that first call to my father upon entering the prison population. My dad told me, *"Son, you've got to take care of yourself. Do whatever you can to get STRONGER, FASTER, and SMARTER. Work out every part of your body, even your fingers if you can. This is now your number one priority as you'll need every advantage possible if you want to survive!"* Needless to say, I took his advice to heart.

Of course in prison your workout options are limited. You can only go to the gym at certain times. There are no free weights, only machines. Food options are limited (no protein powders or GNC stores inside!). So you have to make the best of what you have. That said, at first I wasn't in prison. You see, whenever a person is arrested, he's put into what's often called "county jail." Little did I or my family know at that time, but county jail was far different from what they call "prison." My assumption was that if you're locked up, you're locked up. Why have two separate entities? Turns out, county jail is where the local authorities place people who have not yet been convicted of any crime. In other words, this is where you spend your "innocent until proven guilty" time. So if what I described earlier was prison, you'd think the county would be light-years better, right? Wrong!

During my 19 months in the county lockup, I discovered the harsh reality that the phrase "innocent till proven guilty" is a mythical farce. Good in theory yet nonexistent in reality. This place, this county jail was pure hell. And that's in comparison to prison, a place where I also spent many years. To name a few issues I had with the lockup: you've got no privacy, zero physical contact with your friends and family, grossly negligent health care, a diet fit for a preteen, and nothing that might help you maintain some sort of physical-fitness standard. I couldn't even run. I was trapped with seven slightly psychotic men inside of a concrete box smaller than most family homes. Yep, that means no outside time, either. I literally stepped foot outside TWICE in my first year there. Think about that for a moment. I never missed an opportunity, either. That's all they "took us out."

Take a moment and go, if you would, out to your mailbox and back three times. Seriously, physically get up and go do it. Good, now imagine that is *it* for the next 365 days. Not one single step outside again until this time next year. Congratulations, you've just officially gone outside once more than I did in my first year locked up as a man convicted of absolutely nothing. Welcome to the land of "innocent till proven guilty"! The greatest justice system in the world!!!

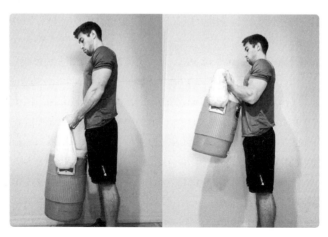

The "Coffee Curl"

The good thing about human beings is that we adapt. The floor became my bench press, the stairs my pull-up bar, a short wall my dip bar, the mat I slept on my sit-up station, and a plastic coffee jug my curl bar. This little patch of enclosed concrete I shared with my new friends was not only my living room, kitchen, dining room, and bedroom, it was also my gym.

For nearly two years, this was all I had. Nothing more, nothing less. Not nearly as much as prison, where convicts get contact visits, food available for purchase, better health care, a touch of privacy, and loads more outdoor time. But it could have been worse. At least that's what I kept trying to tell myself.

It was during my time in the county that I developed my "rudimentary calisthenics" program. Calisthenics? It's a long word with a very simple meaning. Essentially it's working out without equipment or apparatus . . . and that's exactly what I did. Push-ups, pull-ups, sit-ups, dips. You name it, I did it. I even spent hours hitting the concrete walls with my bare fists just to toughen them up. "That sure made for some tough fingers," I thought to myself. **I was going to survive!**

I chose to make the most out of what little I had. That's what I hope this book will do for you . . . show you that it *is* possible. Enough with the excuses. I don't care where you live, what you do, how much space you have, or whether you can afford a gym membership. Those are all convenient mental blocks. *You can still be healthy and in shape no matter where you are in your life.* I did it. So can you.

Okay, so I probably wouldn't recommend punching concrete walls in order to prepare for a fight you hope will never happen. But whatever your circumstances, you know that what I'm saying makes sense. You know the reality. Healthy, attractive people have better opportunities for landing jobs and moving up the social, political, and economic ladder. What's more, the better shape you're in, the better quality of life you will have from the boardroom to the bedroom. Being healthy, fit, and alive just makes sense on every level.

So why put it off? Luckily for you, calisthenics are the perfect starting point. No weights necessary, no running, no gym even. The level of fitness you can achieve through calisthenics alone is astonishing and you can do it anytime, anywhere! Like now for instance. Put down this book and do 10 push-ups and 10 squats. If that's too difficult, it's okay, don't let that bother you. Just try sitting down and getting up five times in a row, or curling your milk jug a few times. Be creative! Come on . . . I mean it. Do it! NOW. Take action!

Just like that you've joined the millions of people doing calisthenics all over the world! How did it feel? Easy, right? That's how I began. I started by alternating workouts every other day in order to build an impressive foundation without doing too much work. Like I said, you can do this anywhere. If you don't feel comfortable going to the gym, that's okay for now. I'll stay home with you and go through these exercises. As stated earlier, they can be done anywhere, right? So, just as I did dips on my bed, you can do them on a chair or any hard surface of similar size. Maybe even do dips off of your bathtub—just make sure the tub's dry! You're only limited by your imagination, the options are limitless!

Instead of using a coffee jug for curls, or for extra weight on squats, you could use a laundry bag or even detergent jugs. Look around. You're surrounded by potential gym equipment. Hopefully you won't have to use these rudimentary objects for long but even if you do, they'll get you started in the right direction. Once you start building that strength and the inner confidence that comes with it, try venturing outside or even to the gym. It all takes time. But go at your own pace while still pushing yourself a bit. It's inevitable, if you keep giving it your best effort, you'll get there.

So here's a bit more of what I did. Now remember there are an endless number of calisthenics routines, which each have their place in the world of fitness, but for now, let's just stick to the basics. If the following workout was enough to make a few hard-core convicts think twice about starting problems with me (and you've seen me), then it should certainly work for you!

Calisthenics

So are you ready to take action? Here's what you do . . . To start, we're going to concentrate on two basic calisthenics exercises: push-ups and squats. Don't know how to do them? It's okay, they're easy. Here are the basic moves . . .

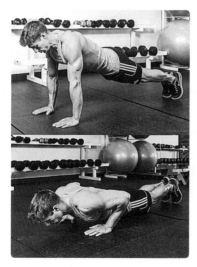

Push-Up

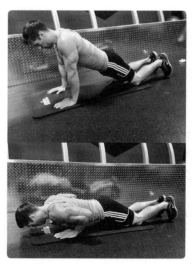

Simple Push-Up Variation

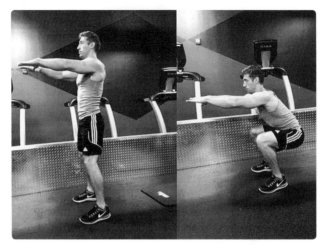

Squat

Okay, now I want you to alternate your basic push-ups and squats, back and forth continuously for 20 minutes with as little rest time in between as possible. Don't worry about how many you can perform, just do as many as you're comfortable with, stopping about one or two reps short of failure, and then take a 15- to 60-second rest before moving on to the next movement. Back and forth, back and forth, back and forth, that's all. It's just that easy and you can do it at home, in the office, in a hotel room, or anywhere you like. Quick note: You may not be able to do nearly as many reps per set at the end of 20 minutes and that's okay, it just means you're doing it right. Below is an example of how the sets and reps of a simple push-up routine might be laid out.

As you can see, getting to 25 push-ups is as simple as doing five sets of five push-ups. You don't have to do five push-ups per set, of course. You don't even have to do five sets. You can change the quantity of these variables to either higher or lower numbers depending on your level of fitness. Just work at your own pace and you're good to go. So long as you feel it, you're improving. All you need for these is the floor and we all have one of these, right?

Sets	Reps
1	5
2	5
3	5
4	5
5	5
5 sets of 5	Total: 25

The next day, try doing some core—think abs—for another 20 or 30 minutes. Switch it up between crunches, planks, and bridges and some stretching. Throw in a few pull-ups, if possible. Do sets of however many crunches you consider appropriate mixed with those bridges and planks, again at whatever number you feel comfortable with. This combo is an ideal workout, since it exercises the main problem areas of your body quickly and effectively. Below are a few workouts that would be a good total core workout. Included are pictures of the moves to guide you through this series of exercises. For starters, it's always good to do three sets of each move at a moderate repetition count: five to 15 reps. Do more of both reps and sets if you can, especially if time allows. This is a great figure-slimming combo that also provides protection in your daily activities. Enjoy!

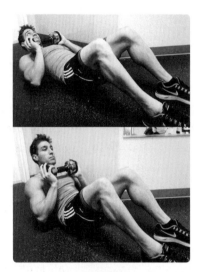

Crunch

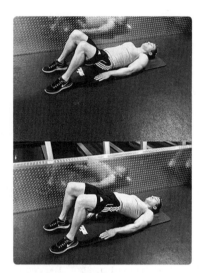

Bridge

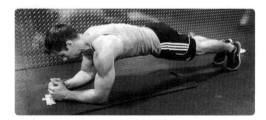

Plank

To Get You Started:

3 sets—crunches

3 sets—bridges

3 sets—planks

Now, this is often when other fitness books will attempt to give some worn-out list of exercises to sound relevant, but that, to me, is missing the point. While I'll detail a few prime workouts in the following pages, I believe it's all about flexibility in your routine and enjoying what you're doing. Just remember to push yourself and to mix it up regarding the body areas you're working. We'll discuss this in further detail a bit later. For now, just remember that it's best not to focus on the same part of your body two days in a row.

Go at your own pace of course, but please try to go as hard as you can on these main moves. It is imperative that you push your limits and build the solid foundation necessary to move forward with your goals. You'll be glad you did!

Now, obviously I was forced into these workouts by my limited options and the fact is that they in and of themselves won't necessarily yield big gains, but don't let this deter you. With the fundamentals down, and a good bit of lean muscle on my frame, I was ready for the weights when the opportunity presented itself. You will be, too.

Before moving along, though, I'd like to stress that these calisthenics movements are not just a warm-up for the big show. To use these valuable tools and subsequently toss them out completely in favor of the weights would be a detriment to your progress. I should know. For many years I did just that.

Upon entering prison for the first time, I had one goal . . . TO GET BIG. I knew nothing about weights, but I did know that guys who had huge muscles (football players, actors, bodybuilders, and the like) got that way by using them. So later on, once I worked out around barbells and such, I ditched my old "friends" (calisthenics) for the tough-guy stuff (weights). And after a bit of time with the weights, I started seeing the gains in strength and size that I'd desired. But something didn't seem quite right. It just seemed as though something was still missing. Basically, the weights did incredibly well at working out individual areas of my body, but calisthenics were what made me feel connected and capable of functioning as one solid unit. Like anything from sports to playing music to writing books, it's important that we never let go of the fundamentals. And going back to these building blocks in everything I've done in life, including my workouts, has always brought about vast improvements.

Honestly, NOT ENOUGH CAN BE SAID ABOUT FUNDAMENTALS. So begin your calisthenics routine now. Get the fundamentals down and move forward, but always come back to what got you going in the first place. Even now, after nearly a decade of weight training, I incorporate at least two days of push-up, pull-up, and body-weight squat exercises into my predominantly power-lifting weekly workouts, and it has left me feeling better than ever. Balance is everything!

As far as I'm concerned, your calisthenics workout can never be too varied; you just have to find what's right for you and your body. Keep in mind, though, that if you want to see specific gains in a certain area of your body, then it's best to concentrate the majority of your reps on the part of the body you're looking to develop. More reps equal more work and more work generally adds up to a bigger, stronger, and more defined body part. Just be sure to give those hard-worked muscles that good rest time they love so much. Balance is key for maximum growth.

Choose Your Moves

As you can imagine, there are countless different calisthenics moves you can use to get started. Listed below are just a few. They are organized by what I consider the five main parts of our body: chest, back, shoulders, legs, and, of course, abs or, more appropriately, the core.

Chest	Back	Shoulders
Decline Push-Up	Pull-Up	Handstand Push-Up w/o Wall
Dip	Inverted Row	Handstand Push-Up w/ Wall
Push-Up	Chin-Up	Handstand Hold w/o Wall
Diamond Push-Up	Superman	Handstand Hold w/ Wall
Explosive Push-Up	Back Extension	Inverted Shoulder Press

Legs	Core
Squat	Plank
Box Jump	Hanging Leg Raise
Pistol Squat	Back Extension
Lunge	Reverse Crunch
Long Jump	Lying Leg Raise
Hip Raise	Regular Crunch
Calf Raise	Side Crunch

I've taken the liberty of presenting these moves in what I consider is the order of importance for each part of the body. So, if performing a leg workout, for example, I would generally use squats and lunges over calf raises. I've also tried to select moves that require no equipment, but I have included a pull-up bar for the back routine and hanging leg raises. There's no way around it, unfortunately, but if you don't have access to a bar that's okay, just skip the majority of the back section for now. For more details of how to perform all of the following moves, as well as why you may want to use them, please refer to the Appendix. For even more practice instructions and detailed visuals, visit my YouTube channel, Ryan Ferguson Fitness.

Two Sample Routines

The primary idea of calisthenics in this book is to lay the foundations for developing a stronger, leaner, and more aesthetically pleasing body. If performed correctly, these exercises will help build what you need to get you into the weight room and on the path to realizing your full potential. They are also all I had for more than a year and a half of my life and *they worked*. These are what I call "no-excuse Prison-Based Routine (PBR) workouts" because they can be done anywhere, at any time. So let's look at two different calisthenics routines that offer both weight-loss and muscle-building potential. The first, as you will see, is faster paced and requires less time. This is good for people on the go, and it also offers a boost to your cardiovascular health while incinerating fat in a way that the other routine may not. The second routine is a little slower paced and may work better for some of you out there (myself included). While less focused on cardiorespiratory enhancement, it does offer a greater opportunity to build the muscular base you'll need in the gym.

Both routines are useful depending on your goals, so I actually tend to mix them up when I can. In fact, I recommend trying both approaches and seeing what works for you. I'll have to warn you, if you're into flashy workouts with lots of variety that will do very little for you, this isn't them. That, in my humble opinion, is why these work. Welcome to the antibullshit PBR workout!

Routine #1: "The Nonconformist"
DURATION: 20 TO 30 MINUTES

This routine is fairly simple. Just perform a few different exercises, including those for the back, legs, and core, for example, and cycle through sets of them over and over again with as little rest time as possible (none, ideally) until you're through. This is one of my favorites! You may not look cool doing it but it'll burn loads of fat while building muscle. For an explanation of the name of this routine read the description for routine #2.

Example: Say I choose pull-ups for my back, lunges for my legs, and regular crunches for my core. My set list would look like the chart on the next page.

Yep, it's that easy! You can change how many reps you perform of each exercise in each set and your rest times but that's about all there is to it. This method, with three exercises in succession, is called a "tri-set." If you performed two exercises, it would be called a "super-set." You can perform a bigger "circuit" with more exercises if you like, but seeing as how I'm not that daring I wouldn't know what to call it. Sorry, but you're on your own there!

Set 1
5 Pull-Ups
5 Lunges
10 Crunches
Rest for 30 seconds
Repeat for 30 minutes

Routine #2: "Prison Pimpin'"

DURATION: 30 TO 60 MINUTES

I like performing this routine outside because it gives me a pump while still providing enough time to relax a little so that I can enjoy the warmth of the sun on my face and the breeze on my skin (weather permitting, of course). A set is generally one exercise at a time, performed to near failure, with a significant rest (30 to 90 seconds) in between. If you're wondering where this name came from, you'd have to see how all the guys in prison act. Most are too cool to actually "work out," so this provides them the opportunity to get the workout they want while not losing that cool factor. That's pimpin', baby! It won't really burn fat, though, or give you any cardio, so that's why you still have to be a "nonconformist."

For this workout, I'm going to give two examples. The first involves an exercise I find very challenging: handstand push-ups against a wall. It's okay if you cannot do these yet. It took me a while to achieve, and it's something for the more advanced readers to begin working toward. If it's too difficult, then substitute with an exercise within calisthenics that focuses on the shoulder, like the inverted shoulder press. That's what's so great about these workouts—they can be mixed and matched to accommodate an array of different body types, skill levels, and goals. Because handstands are so difficult, I would generally perform a low number of reps (like five) while keeping the rest time at a 90-second maximum. If, however, I chose push-ups (an exercise I find quite simple) as in example number two, then I would typically aim for a higher rep count, like 25, while keeping my rest time low—30 to 45 seconds.

Do these moves over and over and over again. That's all there is to it. If you begin getting tired, that's okay. Just perform fewer reps, rest a little longer between sets, and keep at it until your time is up. I've gone down to one handstand push-up or ten regular push-ups during my 60-minute workouts and felt great for completing my workout. It also felt great looking at my gains in the mirror the next day, the next month, and especially the next year. Again, slow and simple yields steady gains. Keep at it and grow!

Example 1	Example 2
SET 1	SET 1
5 Handstand Push-Ups	25 Push-Ups
Rest 60 seconds	Rest 45 seconds
SET 2	SET 2
Repeat set 1 for 30 minutes	Repeat set 1 for 60 minutes

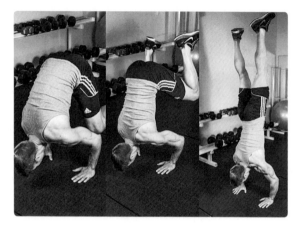

Handstand Push-Up

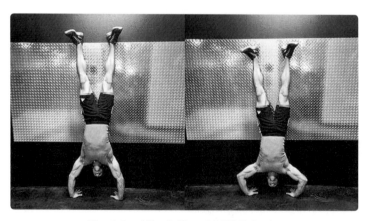

Handstand Push-Up with Wall Assist

The Take

- Calisthenics can be performed anywhere and at any time.
- Sticking to the fundamentals will build strength and improve endurance.
- Performing these workouts can develop a solid foundation for your fitness goals.
- For overall strength gains and balanced growth, keep it varied.
- If you have one specific problem area or muscle you would like to improve, focus more energy (reps, sets, and days) on that specific part of the body.
- Calisthenics can and will help prepare you for weights.

2

If I am through learning, I am through.

—JOHN WOODEN, BASKETBALL COACH

Get Smart

County jail is where I spent the first 19 months of my incarceration. This is the time that passed from the moment I was arrested in March 2004 to my trial, eventual conviction, and sentencing in October 2005. For the first 18 months of this time I had been convicted of absolutely nothing . . . ever. So why didn't I bail out? Logic would dictate that this might have been the wise thing to do. If I had, I could have personally vetted a more appropriate attorney. Beyond that, I could have held a job so that I could afford to pay for this representation. I could have been with my family, had proper medical and dental, been actually innocent till proven guilty . . . the list goes on. Who wouldn't want to bail out? It seems so simple. I mean, it says right there in the Eighth Amendment of the Constitution that "Excessive bail shall not be required, nor excessive fines imposed, nor cruel and unusual punishments inflicted."

Unfortunately, the reality was that I never had a legitimate chance to bail out. This also means that I never got a chance for all of those things we take for granted like seeing a dentist, working to support myself, and having the opportunity to research attorneys, while being accused of a crime I had absolutely nothing to do with. The reason for all of this . . . the astonishing and, in my opinion, the "excessive" $20 million bail, by far the largest of its kind historically, that was so kindly given to me by the "honorable" Judge Ellen Roper. No record, no priors, NO COMMON SENSE. Nonetheless, with no accountability for the individuals making these decisions, this was my reality, and regardless of what was right or wrong, I had to make the best of it.

That's why, during this hellish period, calisthenics served an incredibly important role. But I quickly realized that these workouts alone would not create the body necessary to survive prison. Going from the county jail (where your foes are essentially emaciated, helpless, deprived shells of themselves) to prison (where pure, unharnessed hate runs deep) is like the difference between the peewee league and the pros.

These people, these seasoned vets of the penitentiary game, were the real deal. These were the true convicts, those who had been plotting and scheming in this strange, twisted environment for years—in many cases longer than I'd even been alive. It's here that you face the reality of prison life: the cold walls, razor wire, and oppressive confinement of a tiny concrete box. This is their existence, and you quickly come to realize that, while many of these inmates may never leave prison, they do occasionally get to leave their cells. And when they do, anything can happen. A wayward look, one single misstep, the slightest misunderstood word, and all hell can break loose. Your life can be forever altered in the blink of an eye.

I've seen it happen all too often. My first memory of such an event in prison was when this guy I rode in on the bus with, we'll call him Peter, began getting picked on. To this day I still don't know why it happened but I'm almost certain it was unprovoked. He was just standing in line at the chow hall and this rather largish nut decided to throw his lit cigarette at Peter's back. Peter chose to do nothing, so the nut bends down, picks up the cigarette, and then proceeds to throw it at Peter's face. Once again Peter does nothing. Then this guy leans in and whispers something to Peter. That was it. No overt violence. No big scene. Nothing.

Later that day, though, I see the nutty guy walk up to Peter's cell and take all his food and smokes while Peter idly watches. This was not exactly a transaction done out of the goodness of Peter's heart. From that day forth, Peter never had any respect. People took whatever they wanted from him and treated him like a pariah. Needless to say, Peter's time in prison was very difficult. One small, cowardly move like the one from Peter, and the next 20 years of life becomes exponentially more difficult.

While this story may not seem incredibly graphic, I can assure you, worse things were going on behind the scenes when those weirdos ventured into Peter's cell. This was quite a common outcome for the weak, pathetic men who lacked the physical or mental capacity to stand up for themselves. Over the years I'd see this scenario play out time and time again. This is what I'd refer to as the passive form of physical dominance, and to me, it was far scarier than the other spurts of more overt, more severe violence.

Remember, Peter's experience was just my first encounter with the games people play in prison. I've seen multiple people get stabbed over less than $50 of bad dope they weren't willing to pay for, jaws broke over cutting ahead of people in the chow line, compliments of an old acquaintance from the county jail. Glad I never pissed him off. And worst of all, I had to listen to a man get beat damn near to death while screaming for help. All over a disagreement about who would get to yell out the door to their buddies. We were locked down all day in "the hole," and this was our only form of communication. Apparently they both had something important to say.

As you can imagine, no one is safe in prison. But you quickly learn that the new, the weak, and the ignorant are the most vulnerable. In prison the saying "only the strong survive" is frighteningly accurate. These words no longer applied to winning in sports or making good grades as they once did in my youth. Gritty and raw though they may be, these words now applied to my very existence, my survival, *my life*. This game has no pause, no reset, and it certainly had no extra lives.

Now it was my turn. "Fight or flight, little buddy?" For me, though, there really was no choice. *Fight!* It's who I am. It's who I've always been and who I'll always be. The only problem is . . . I can't fight. That, and the fact that these guys were BIG! Not only were they big but they were bad. All I could think was: "What am I doing here?"

So when I caught my first glimpse of the weights in prison, I was ecstatic. I was small, even more so than I'd realized, and I knew this pile of iron was my only hope. No one could help me anymore and those weights offered me . . . POWER! Now, if I could only figure out how to use the damn things before time ran out.

I remember thinking to myself, "How difficult can this be?" Fact is, I was young and athletic so I figured all I needed to do was hit the gym, knock out a few bench presses, do some curls, and voilà, I'd be in Schwarzenegger shape before I knew it! I'd attempted lifting weights for about a month while in college, but as we all know, my college career hit an abrupt end. Sad really, as I think I would have excelled where I was at. Good gym, good roomie, good school. It all just felt so right . . .

Anyway, aided by this frame of mind and my completely useless month of working out two years prior, I went into the gym with zero plan of action. All I told myself was "Push all the weight you can, little buddy," and that's exactly what I did. It worked, too . . . for a while. As the days and weeks slowly rolled by without too frightening an incident, I enjoyed a few slight gains but nowhere near what I'd hoped for, especially given the incredible effort I'd been putting in. That's how I learned what is probably the most important lesson in weight training: IT TAKES BRAINS!!!

While growing up, I heard people make fun of, or at the very least, talk down to "meatheads." For those not in the know about this particular name, in very loose terms meatheads are the guys who are presumably large in muscle while significantly lacking in mental mass. This is where my buddy Sam comes in. Maybe it was because of his build or maybe it was because he came off as a bully, but the embarrassing fact is that I chose to call him this name once during a rather comical debate. I guess words were my only weapon since he was twice my size, and I, quite simply, had nothing else to fight back with. How creative, right?

Anyway, long story short . . . it didn't work. Sam got pissed and used those gigantic arms of his to push me about six feet through the air, flat onto my backside. Needless to say, it wasn't a mistake I would be making again! I would later find out, after we'd reconciled our differences, that this guy was actually pretty intelligent. He had a decent vocabulary, kept up on current events, and even read quite a bit. Looking back now, it is obvious who the real "meathead" was.

Little did I know then that this experience would later come in handy as I adjusted to prison life full time. For almost two years I had been on lockdown 24 hours a day at the county jail. During this time I'd educated myself on such things as politics, vocabulary, and literature with great success. Now I knew it was time to get smart about my body. So I decided to marry my mind and my muscle in an effort to maintain what little power I still possessed over my life.

It turned out to be a pivotal decision and one that forever altered my life in numerous ways. Knowledge is the golden ticket! That's why the rich and famous have personal trainers. It can take years of time, energy, and dedication to sort through all the garbage out there. Almost everyone who is in good shape can tell you stories of their setbacks: the mistakes they made, the diets that failed, and the resolutions they broke. I have a feeling many of you reading this book know exactly what I'm talking about. It takes time to sift through all the nonsense out there when it comes to training, and sadly, time is something I had a lot of. So here is years' worth of info right at your fingertips. All accessible within hours. That is, of course, a major reason for writing this book.

But why do so many people go so wrong when it comes to working out and maintaining a healthy lifestyle? I think there are two main causes: information overload and isolationist training.

INFORMATION OVERLOAD: Head to any bookstore or surf the exercise and fitness books section of Amazon, and you'll soon experience plenty of this! Sadly, information overload is an issue that stops many people dead in their tracks. It can take years to distinguish the fluff from the fundamentals. As a result, many people don't know where to start and ultimately become disillusioned. As I said earlier, that is why this book exists. Just follow the few basic rules here, put in a little hard work, dedicate yourself to what you know works, and the rest just comes with time. No magic bullet, no fads, and certainly no "diets."

Once you've read through this book and adopted the fundamentals, I believe your future reading in this area will become much more productive. You'll know what the writers are talking about, why the article exists, and how to get to the meat of what's being said. A lot of what's written is just crap to fill the pages—there is not a whole lot of new, groundbreaking knowledge out there. That said, I'm constantly coming across little tidbits that reveal themselves every once in a while. Just remember to let the inconsistencies and contradictions go. There are still loads of useful info in these sources, and the more you read, the more you understand. It'll get easier to find what you need, I promise.

ISOLATIONIST TRAINING: They say variety is the spice of life and when it comes to health and fitness, I wholeheartedly agree! Too often people try to attain their physical goals from one isolated angle. The unfortunate reality is that this will never work.

You *need* a multifaceted approach to health if you hope to ever succeed. Diet, exercise, cardio, weight training, and even rest and recovery are all spokes in the same wheel of total body fitness. They are ALL essential ingredients, and without a healthy dose of each, along with balance, your progress will be limited. If you love banging out the big weights or curling your body into a pretzel in a yoga class that's great. But don't let that be the sum total of your approach to fitness. You have to mix it up.

Knowing there are so many aspects to cover in your fitness regimen may at first seem quite daunting. Without knowing it, however, you've already taken one of the biggest steps toward conquering your goals. Understanding and accepting that there are NO simple, quick, or gimmicky solutions to sustained physical prowess IS the first step. The more you educate yourself, the quicker you'll achieve the body of your dreams. That's the real shortcut.

Unfortunately, without this core logic, many individuals, myself included, have ended up wasting time and energy without understanding why. So once again, just as in Chapter 1, it's time to make a choice. Get smart and get fit or continue to make easily avoidable mistakes. My friends, it's up to you. As Bush Jr. might say, you are the "decider" of your fate. The future is in your hands.

So what's next, you may be thinking? More awareness of course! While it may sound like a bit of a bore to have to spend more time in the classroom, please allow me to share one little secret with you. Due to my willingness to invest a little time up front studying the secrets of a healthier diet and advanced fitness principles, I was able to spend the rest of my days being "lazy" while still enjoying incredible gains. Meanwhile, many of my fellow inmates ended up working twice as hard with nothing to show for their efforts.

Our bodies work in very measurable, highly predictable ways. As you will see again and again throughout this book, the importance of planning is paramount. A certain type of workout, the proper form of cardio, even something as simple as eating at the right times all deliver tried and tested results. The secrets are all out there. You just have to do your research, which starts here! Remember, I was trapped in a concrete box with very few resources for almost 10 years of my life. Many of you, on the other hand, have the world at your fingertips. All you need is just a few keyboard clicks away! There are no excuses.

What's more is that once you've gained this awareness and made these small changes, you'll continue with them for life. "When you know better, you do better," as the saying goes.

Knowledge only becomes power when it's actually USED! That is the essence of why I wrote this book . . . so I could put the proverbial ball back in your court. I'm sharing all the lessons I've worked so hard to learn over this past decade in one simple book, so that YOU, and only YOU, can control your destiny. NO MORE EXCUSES. The more changes you make, the greater your success will be.

NOTE: While this book contains everything I believe is necessary to begin heading down the path to better health, a better body, and ultimately a better quality of life, there are endless possibilities of things you may also find beneficial. That's why I continue to educate myself: I'm positive there are always MORE lessons to be learned.

That said, I must also stress how important it is that you take control of this continued, lifelong self-education. We are all unique and you'll be amazed at what you may find helpful, which someone else may have overlooked. I've discovered this multiple times, as my friends have come up with all types of amazing things that I might never have noticed. We can ALWAYS learn more and we can ALWAYS be better. Remember . . . GROW YOUR MIND, GROW YOUR BODY!

The Take

- Getting into shape takes a serious commitment to obtaining knowledge.
- Making small investments of time to learn now can pay dividends for a lifetime.
- Save time and energy by learning about your diet and the best ways to work out.
- Read everything you can get your hands on, including (but not limited to) nutrition books, workout books, magazines, newspapers, studies, reports, and fitness websites. Not all of them will be great and some will undoubtedly contradict others, but if you can learn at least one helpful tip from each, your goals will be that much more attainable.
- Try out what you read and see if it works for your body type and your needs.
- Remember: getting the body you desire requires a multifaceted approach.
- Working out smart and eating right allow you to be "lazy."

- Make small, manageable changes.
- Keep in mind that no matter how much you think you know, there's always more to learn.
- Knowledge gives you the power to create the body you want.

SO WHAT ARE YOU WAITING FOR? TAKE ACTION!

3

*Rowing harder doesn't help if the boat
is headed in the wrong direction.*

—KENICHI OHMAE

The Big Six Moves

Fall 2005. After almost two years of being locked away from my family in what can only be described as a massive stack of cinder block, it was time for the next stage of my physical development. Getting big in a hurry. The reason: my life depended on it. In prison the stakes are truly life and death. Here's an example.

One day I was preparing to go to the gym when I became aware of a "code red," high alert. Cops were running, lights were flashing, and COs (corrections officers) were yelling at us to lock down immediately! Something was happening and it felt big.

Now, in prison, getting locked down from time to time isn't a big deal. But this one was different. The timing was off, the actions of the authorities were strange, and EVERYONE was sent back inside their cells. That was a bit unusual. I didn't know what to make of it.

Two and a half hours later, with no word as to what was going on (we were usually left in the dark), normal movement was back and all was fine . . . kind of. It was 6:30 p.m. and I was due to be at work tutoring other inmates. Something I greatly enjoyed volunteering for as it helped others attain their GEDs. On this night, though, I didn't want to be there. I didn't want to leave my cell. Things just felt a bit *off.* It was as if the administration was *trying* to be normal. Instead . . . it just felt spooky. You see, prison is a strange little world where word often travels fast. Sure enough, on my arrival at school, everyone was talking about that afternoon's incident, a brutal murder that had supposedly occurred in the house next to mine, Six House. Not that a murder in prison was uncommon. When you force two strangers to live together in a 10 × 10 concrete box, and one, the other, or both are killers or, at the very least, criminally violent lunatics, you can figure out what might happen. In this case the murderer had beaten his cellmate to near death and stuffed his body under the bunk to die a lonely, terrifying, slow, and painful death.

At the time, my immediate thought was, "That could have been me." And the frightening reality was: this almost *was* me, multiple times. Seven House ("the hole") was bad, and Six House, a "better part of the hole," was far worse. Thankfully, toward the end of my imprisonment I was in Five House, right next door but worlds away in terms of mentality, violence, and stress levels. This wasn't by accident, either. I worked hard to get into this housing unit and even harder to stay there.

In short, I had to endure a yearlong intense program where my life was essentially under the control of the administrators. We marched, went to classes and group sessions from five in the morning to nine at night, got five minutes to shower, and followed more rules than could fit into this book. It was crazy, but still a good thing. I believe it's actually even helped a few people. If only prison focused more on simple solutions to *correcting* people's bad habits and behaviors than locking them in a box for years on end, then it's possible that some good would come out of the incarceration part of our justice system.

Anyway, this living situation hadn't always been an option. Years earlier I was forced to share a tiny cell in those obscenely oppressive housing units with a bizarre mix of random psychopaths, everyone from carjackers to robbers to merciless killers. Some were smaller than I was, most were larger, but ALL were undoubtedly crazier, and in prison, that's what you've really got to watch out for: the nuts. So when I heard about this brutal murder, all I could think was the next time it could well be me stuffed under that bunk. I was struck by a moment of total and complete panic. The reality is, as long as you're stuck in prison, you just never know what might happen next.

Which brings me back to the beginning of my prison journey. My first celly in a maximum-security prison was Markis. He was one bad dude. In prison for robbing dope houses in Kansas City, Markis was a seasoned vet. Prison was his second home and, by all accounts, this was his world. Fortunately, Markis and I got along . . . most of the time. Not good but well enough to keep the peace. I'd like to say the peacekeeping was mutual, but to be honest, it was mainly due to my grudging acceptance of the things I could not control or change (primarily his massive size and intimidating demeanor). Needless to say, I had to make many frustrating concessions. Wipe down the sink and leave it looking pristine (he was OCD). Read facing the wall instead of out toward the room (his paranoia told him I was watching his every move). Don't breathe too loud. (Apparently I did this on purpose? A complaint I'd never heard prior to or after this nut.) The list goes on. I'd love to say I did it simply because I was the "bigger man," which I was inside, but my choices were slim, and he was without a doubt the *bigger man* in that cell.

At six feet three inches tall, packed with 230 pounds of pure muscle, and covered from head to toe in demonic tattoos, made all the more intimidating by the scars from the shotgun blast that had rearranged the upper left side of his face and body, this guy was not someone I wanted to have problems with. Especially not while I was trapped in our temporary concrete cage, where help may as well have been miles away. Worse still, my new "friend" Markis had been medically diagnosed with bipolar disorder and rediagnosed by me to be totally and completely freakin' delusional.

Yep, if there ever was a welcoming committee to prison, it would be this guy. I hated to admit it, but I was powerless. This guy may as well have been Mike Tyson standing in front of me. All I knew was: (1) I was way too small to deal with this guy; (2) I'd fight to the death if this guy tried anything (not like it'd be much of a fight but I really had no choice in the matter); and (3) well, he knew 1 and 2. Right away I knew my first three months in prison were guaranteed to be interesting.

The silver lining to this situation, if there was one, was that Markis worked out hard, and knowing this helped motivate me to do the same. Not necessarily because I wanted to, but because I *had* to. Living with an unstable individual like Markis, danger was always right around the corner, so it was in my best interest to "keep up." I use the phrase "keeping up" quite loosely because even after ten years of dedicating myself to fitness, I still can't necessarily say that I'm all the way caught up. Fact: you can't beat crazy!

I came to realize quite quickly that my single most imminent danger was not, as I had thought, out on the yard around all of the crazies, thugs, and creeps, but rather in what should be my "safe zone," locked up with a madman behind an impenetrable steel door, with nowhere to run. Trapped like a rat with the craziest, baddest people on earth. Help would never come. It's you against psycho roid rage over there and that's it. Battle royal, baby, a fight to the end.

So while I had made modest gains at first, gains that most people would have been proud of, I still had a long way to go. Staring at the image in the mirror, all I could think was: "Who's going to be afraid of your skinny little ass?" So I ate more, I worked out harder, and I hit the books.

Ultimately, I came to realize that much of what I'd been spending my time on in the gym was quite useless. Lesson #1: All workouts are NOT created equal. Things really began to change for me when I learned this important lesson.

My breakthrough came when I learned about compound moves, the basis of this chapter. Now there are many compound moves out there, but we're interested primarily in what I consider the Big Six: the squat, deadlift, pull-עup, bent-over row, bench press, and shoulder press.

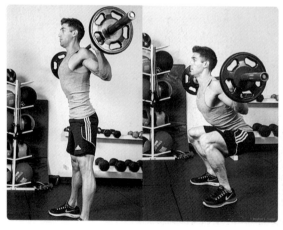

Legs: Squat

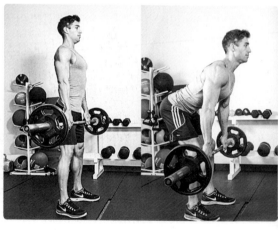

Legs: Deadlift

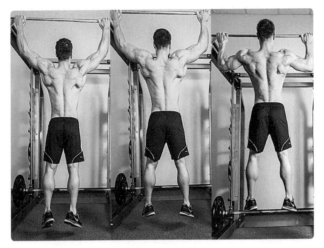

Back: Pull-Up

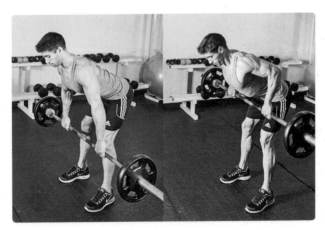

Back: Bent-Over Row

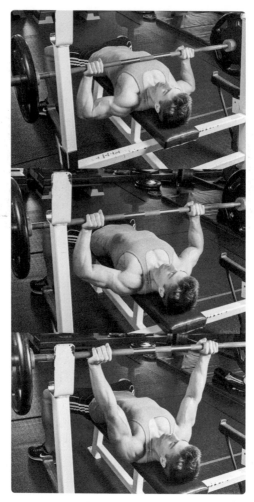

Chest: Bench Press

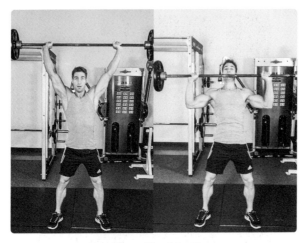

Shoulders: Shoulder Press

The Big Six

There are four general areas of the body these six main moves work: the chest, the back, the shoulders, and the all-important legs. (Your abs—core—have their own chapter, Chapter 7, but it's important to note that all the moves in this chapter stimulate the core.) These moves can be arranged in a variety of ways, depending on your workout's time constraint and goals. This list is broken down by areas of the body so that you can visualize where to best fit these exercises into your routine. While there is no right or wrong regimen per se, I generally stick to two or three main moves a day (along with my interchangeable exercises) and keep them in the same or opposing families (legs with legs or back with back).

There are quite a few reasons for not using all six moves at once, but the main two for me are time and quality constraints. In order to target each muscle properly, it would take a larger chunk of time than most people have available. Even if you could fit it all in, the quality of your workouts would likely diminish due to reduced energy levels. Not only this, but you would then be forced to take a rest day after every day of working out, thus severely limiting your *quality gym time.* That's why I advise concentrating on two or three areas a day, so that you'll always leave yourself more to do the next workout session while avoiding overtraining and ultimately seeing better gains.

If performed correctly, these compound, or multijoint, moves will provide you with far more gains than isolated movements (single-joint movements) and will do so in significantly less time. In fact, if these compound movements are the only exercises you ever do, you'll still be light-years ahead of your friends. Here's why: While isolation movements such as curls, skull crushers, calf raises, or almost any exercise performed on a machine put the focus on a single muscle or group of muscles, often without the use of smaller stabilizing muscles, multijoint moves vastly expand your workload by forcing multiple areas of your body to work in unison.

For example, take the king of exercises, the squat. With the weight on your shoulders, you bend your knees, activating the obvious muscles: hams, quads, and glutes. But while these muscles, some of the largest in the body, are the primary focus of the squat, the benefits don't end there. In fact, studies have shown that squats activate approximately 250 individual muscles. The reason? While you're squatting, you're forcing all types of smaller stabilizing muscles in your core, hips, back, and legs to keep your body properly aligned. So, faced with a choice between performing quad extensions, which work just one tiny group of muscles, or a squat, the choice is obvious.

There's more good news! As you probably know, there's a direct correlation between the amount of muscle you actually work and calories burned. So by using compound movements, you're burning far more calories in less time. Who wouldn't love that?

Want more? Not only do you burn more calories in less time while performing compound movements, these exercises also activate your metabolism. The result, you burn even MORE calories long after you've finished your workout. The reason, which we'll cover in greater depth later, is that once you've broken down your muscles in the gym, they need to repair themselves outside of the gym (a.k.a. the "growth phase"). This process requires energy, often in the form of . . . calories. MORE MUSCLES IN NEED OF REPAIR = MORE CALORIES BURNED.

It also means bigger, stronger, and faster muscles, all while you sit on the couch watching the duck people, *The Bachelor*, or whatever people get into these days. Need I say more?

Okay, here's one final advantage. All the extra muscle mass you gain by performing compound exercises over other, less effective exercises pays one last, never-ending dividend. The more lean muscle mass you carry around, the more calories you burn in a sedentary state. This means that even if you don't work out, you'll still be burning more calories watching TV than the person sitting next to you. So what are you waiting for? Build and burn! Start using the Big Six Moves now!

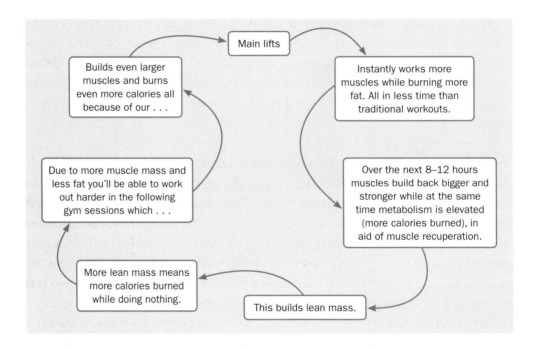

Muscle Confusion—Why Not ALL Change Is Good

As you can see, all you have to do is stick to these tried-and-tested lifts. Your workout doesn't have to be too sexy or nearly as exotic as many people often assume. In fact, I'd strongly suggest NOT getting too exotic. These Big Six movements are scientifically proven to use the most muscle fibers at one time, meaning more work is being accomplished in less time. You're growing more muscle, burning more calories, and boosting your metabolism all at once. THIS IS THE KEY to unlocking your potential in the gym.

What's more, you can stick to, and gain from, these same basic movements for a lifetime. Whether you've been working out for years or are a complete novice when it comes to weights, I'm sure you've likely heard of the importance of "muscle confusion." The basic idea is that if you follow the same workouts time and again your body will eventually get used to the movements and your gains will plateau. Unfortunately, the problem with this concept is that, more often than not, it causes "MENTAL CONFUSION."

This is because most people don't really understand the concept of "muscle confusion." It's not their fault, though. I blame it on many of the outlandish books and magazines out there. The most common misinterpretation is that you should periodically, every six to 12 weeks, change up the exercises you are performing. NOT TRUE. Too often people end up swapping up their routines just as they're about to make some significant gains! In my opinion, you should ALWAYS incorporate these Big Six Moves into your workouts and add anything else that you feel has worked well for your specific body type and has garnered positive results.

Now, that's not to say that no change is necessary. Often all that's needed is a little tweaking here and there, every now and then. This can be done in a multitude of ways: by changing the amount of weight you're using (heavy or light); the amount of reps you perform (ranging anywhere from one all the way up to 100); or by doing something as simple as switching up the order of your workout by prefatiguing (placing more emphasis on the muscle group you're most interested in targeting).

Whatever route you take, there will inevitably be endless ways to switch up your workout, but you've got to stick to the essentials. Just as you can't win a basketball game without shooting the basketball, you can't develop your legs, build your core, or get a nice butt without doing squats.

Keep It Casual

Finally, I want to stress the importance of "keeping it casual" during all of your workouts. While there's a time and a place for precisely regimented workouts—the type you'll find in most books and magazines—my belief is that these hard-core programs aren't strictly necessary for the average person. Personally, I want to look and feel good, but I don't want the journey getting there to feel like a trip through Dante's inferno! In my experience, and from the people I've helped meet their goals, I've found that if you make your workout enjoyable, you'll end up working harder, feeling better, and wanting to come back for more.

So my preference is to have a semistructured workout plan that leaves a few things open to chance and feeling. Now some of you may prefer a highly regimented program, but I find some looseness helps me stay mentally focused and avoid burnout. It also prevents boredom and enables you to "listen" to your body. As long as you stick to the Big Six Moves, then everything else can be fun and slightly improvised.

The programs I outline in this chapter feature a mix of the Big Six Moves and your own interchangeable moves. You're going to perform the latter after you've worked those all-important multijoint lifts. These interchangeable moves can be added, dropped, or moved around to hit specific areas of your body, thus rounding out your workout and keeping you well-balanced without losing interest in what would otherwise be the same old routine. As you've probably already noticed, there's yet another benefit to not being so regimented: *real* muscle confusion! By using this technique, your muscles won't know what to expect next and growth will be inevitable!

One final note. "Keeping it casual" does not mean going to the gym to socialize or text your friends while you're on the bench press (sound like anyone you know?). It's simply referring to a relaxed workout structure, so no excuses. GO HARD!!!

Interchangeable Moves

Okay, here are those promised secondary moves! As you can see, I've broken down the list into the same four categories as the Big Six above. Simply take two or three interchangeable moves from the same muscle group as Big Six Moves and start building your workout. In general, I like to use about six exercises per workout—two Big Six Moves and four interchangeable moves. I then complete about five sets per exercise for a total of 30 sets.

The best part—my workouts never get stale, since I'm constantly changing up the routine!

See the Appendix for details on each move and check out my YouTube page, Ryan Ferguson Fitness, for step-by-step instructional videos.

Back
Inverted Row
Lateral Pull-Down
Crossover Rear Lateral Raise
Cable Row
Back Extensions

Shoulders
Dumbbell Shoulder Press
Dumbbell or Cable Front Raise
Dumbbell or Cable Side Raise
Shrug
Bent-Over Dumbbell Raise

Legs
Box Jump
Sled Push
Leg Curl
Leg Extension
Dumbbell Step-Up
Weighted Step-Up
Weighted Lunge
Calf Raises

Chest
Dip
Dumbbell Fly
Cable Fly

Arms	
Biceps	Barbell Curl
	Reverse Curl
	Hammer Curl
Forearms	Wrist Curl
	Wrist Extension
	Pull-Up Hold
Triceps	Close Grip Bench
	Skull Crusher
	Tri Push-Down with Bar
	Tri Push-Down with Rope
	Single Arm Press-Down

Sample Plans

Ready to get to work? Below I've outlined two different routines, a three-day-a-week workout plan and a six-day plan for those of you who just can't wait to hit the iron!

Again, feel free to modify these plans based on your lifestyle, schedule, and how much cardio you want to utilize in your workouts. Keeping it fresh and appropriate for your changing needs is the name of the game. Keep in mind, these are just sample plans. I don't do the same routine week after week, I constantly shake it up! Nonetheless, I've been utilizing varieties of these workouts for the better part of six years now and continue to see gains that boggle my mind.

This workout burns fat, builds muscle, strengthens the core, gives me a pump, and, most important, leaves me feeling good! I prefer the six-day schedule because I can usually get in and out of the gym in about 30 to 45 minutes. The three-day workouts tend to be a bit longer, since you have to cram more in to engage each part of the body every week, but it's proven useful for those weeks where I've been too busy to go to the gym daily. It also means working out every other day, which is a nice change sometimes. Try both and see what works for you.

So without further ado, here's what I do on a weekly basis. Scratch that, here's what I do for LIFE!

Note: On all workouts for both schedules, lift however much weight you feel comfortable with to reach the number of listed reps while staying about a rep or two away from failure.

Three-Day Workout

DAY 1—LEGS AND SHOULDERS

Exercise	Sets	Reps
Back Squat	3	10
Front Squat	2	10
Shoulder Press (sitting)	5	10
Leg Curl	5	10
Leg Extension	5	10
Shrug	5	10
Cardio 5-minute warm-up	5	20-second intervals

DAY 2—BACK

Exercise	Sets	Reps
Bent-Over Row	5	10
Pull-Up	5	10
Inverted Row	5	10
Cable Row	5	10
Barbell Curl	5	10
Reverse Curl	5	10
Core—see Chapter 7 for abs		

DAY 3—CHEST AND LEGS

Exercise	Sets	Reps
Regular Deadlift	3	10
Straight Leg Deadlift	2	10
Bench Press	5	10
Close Grip Bench	5	10
Dip	5	10
Cable Fly	5	10
Tri Push-Down	5	10
Cardio	5	20-second intervals

Six-Day Work Out

DAY 1—BACK AND SHOULDERS

Exercise	Sets	Reps
Regular Deadlift	5	10
Straight Leg Deadlift	5	10
Back Extensions	5	10
Shoulder Press (standing)	5	10
Bent-Over Dumbbell Raise	5	10
Dumbbell Side Raise	5	10

DAY 2—ABS, INTERVALS, AND BICEPS

Exercise	Sets	Reps
See Chapter 7 for abs		
Dumbbell Curl	5	10
Reverse Grip Barbell Curl	5	10
Hammer Curl with Rope	5	10
Forearm Wrist Curl	5	10
Forearm Wrist Extension	5	10
Cardio Interval 5-minute warm-up and cooldown	10	20 seconds w/ 40 seconds of rest

DAY 3—BACK AND CHEST

Exercise	Sets	Reps
Bent-Over Row	5	10
Bench Press	5	10
Weighted Pull-Up	5	5
Cable Fly	5	10
Cable Row	5	10

DAY 4—ABS, INTERVALS, AND TRICEPS

Exercise	Sets	Reps
See Chapter 7 for abs		
Close Grip Bench	2	10
Tri Push-Down with Bar	5	10
Single Arm Press-Down	5	10
Forearm Wrist Curl	5	10
Forearm Wrist Extension	5	10

DAY 5—LEGS

Exercise	Sets	Reps
Back Squat	5	10
Front Squat	5	10
Leg Press	5	10
Weighted Lunge	5	10
Calf Raise	5	10

DAY 6—ABS AND CARDIO

Exercise
See Chapter 7, abs
30-60-60 minutes steady-state cardio

The Take

- It's possible to build more muscle in less time by using compound moves—especially the Big Six Moves.
- Making compound moves the core of your workout program builds muscle and burns fat better than exercises that target specific body parts.
- Keep workouts clutter-free and simple.
- More muscles worked = more calories burned.
- Compound moves can boost your postworkout metabolism.
- The more lean muscle mass you build, the more calories you burn while in a sedentary state.
- Using compound moves consistently week in, week out builds strength, size, and better body composition.
- Keep your workouts "casual." Don't overstructure your programs.
- Be sure to keep your routine fresh. Rotate those small tweaks in and out every six to eight weeks for sustained growth—but maintain your compound moves.
- Find a regimen you like and that works, and STICK TO IT!

4

I wanna live.

—MY CELLY'S DRY RESPONSE WHEN
ASKED WHY HE RAN SO MUCH

Cardio

Confession time. I've always had a love/hate affair when it comes to cardio and something tells me I'm not alone. Most people fall into one of these two camps. I just happen to feel both ways!

Here's the deal. I love how cardio can dramatically transform your body, making it leaner, more agile, and better defined. Who wouldn't love that? On the other hand, I hate cardio for pretty much every other conceivable reason known to mankind, as well as a few others yet to be discovered!

When I first arrived at prison, cardio was of little concern to me. I needed size, not health, and running around burning the precious few calories I could accumulate was not in my best interest. If the prison population were to compose a menu of potential victims, small, preppy guys much like myself would likely be the main course. Needless to say, I didn't want to do anything that might make me even more of a target. So early on I avoided cardio at all costs.

Unfortunately, I soon reached a point in prison where I couldn't just keep stuffing my face and getting as big as possible, no matter how much I might have wanted to. My body simply couldn't take it any longer. Also, after a few years of navigation through that world, I felt a bit safer from the various predators that lurked, largely due to my increased size and the knowledge I'd gained from prison experience. At the same time, I was also slower, lazier, and lacking the energy necessary to keep up with the torments of prison life. I realized I had to find a balance. And that's where cardio entered my life.

Fortunately for me, as my waistline grew, so did my reputation. I was big and bad. Well . . . not so much on the whole bad thing, but I was generally accepted by the tougher crowd in prison. Why? To this day, I still don't quite know and I sure wasn't going to ask questions. I just accepted this blessing.

People didn't really know what to think of me. I was focused, educated, quiet, and covered in muscle. A good combination, it turns out, for having people leave you alone. For now, I continue to thank the heavens that my fellow inmates didn't know how truly afraid I was. Every moment of every day I felt as though things could go south at any time. I was petrified I'd mess up and my true, slightly less brave colors would be on full display. Once my secret was out . . . well, I dreaded what the consequences might be.

So having reached the apex of my accumulation of mass, I realized it was time to begin the process of turning my unsculpted heap of muscle into something more useful and aesthetically pleasing. It's here that my feelings for cardio turned from dislike into absolute disgust. The beefed-up hulk of a man I'd worked so hard to turn myself into over the course of the past two years couldn't even make it on a three-mile jog without cramping up, feeling wobbly, and getting those dreaded shin splints. My balloon had officially deflated. Turns out, I wasn't anywhere near the enhanced physical specimen I thought I was . . . back to square one.

My thinking was to give it one summer. Cardio, they say (whoever "they" are), is primarily a matter of mental fortitude. If you can push through the growing pains and make it a habit, you will inevitably see incredible results. So I pushed, forcing myself to run three to five miles every other day alongside other cardio activities such as basketball or badminton. One bonus I gained from those runs was peace. After having spent more than a year and a half in what may as well have been a cave, the new outdoor gravel track around the baseball field felt like freedom. I still think about how beautiful those morning runs were. The quiet breeze against my skin coupled with the warmth of the early sun. Plus, most people weren't up that early so I had the track to myself! Too bad that couldn't last longer. As with all good things in prison, administration took that joy away after only a few short summers. What's interesting was I ran for a reason quite foreign to the prison population in general. I was running . . . to keep up my looks.

At this particular point in time, I had an incredibly important hearing coming up and larger media opportunities were looming. While giving interviews is not something I enjoy or will ever really be fully comfortable with, I basically had no choice. As far as I was concerned, the courts were no longer interested in seeking justice, and these TV shows would hopefully provide some level of accountability and bring awareness to the masses. In other words, once again I had to stand up and fight for myself, put myself out there, and beg for people to look at the facts.

Contrary to popular belief, we never initiated contact with programs such as *48 Hours* and *Dateline*. Although I greatly respect these shows' professionalism and the work they did, the reality is that they call you up and essentially say,

"We're going to run a story on your case. Would you like to do an interview?" Regardless of the answer, the show WILL go on. Such is the nature of the beast. So . . . I'd rather say my two cents, thank you very much . . . and hopefully look damn good doing it. This wasn't some interview done for fun, this was my life I was fighting for.

So I ran. The whole time I focused on my survival. I thought about how I would look and come across to a judgmental TV audience. It was these thoughts that kept me going during difficult days when I constantly thought of quitting. Thankfully, over time, I started to build a little momentum in my training. My stamina improved, making the runs easier each week, and I was feeling, as well as seeing, results.

For the first time in my life, I could actually claim to be a runner. I finally knew what it was to push through the runs, fight a mind that's constantly telling you to give in, and ultimately reach that point of bliss where running becomes almost meditative. ALMOST! At times, getting myself out there to run after a hard workout or a tiring day was exceedingly difficult, but those were the days that meant the most to me. These were the days that separated me from the herd.

Having finally battled and conquered cardio, I felt on top of the world. With my diet, workout, and new cardio program now firing on all cylinders, nothing could stop me. I was a machine! Then a week before my birthday and going into the cold months, I severely sprained my ankle in a game of pickup basketball, effectively knocking me out of commission for four months. For three of those months I couldn't even walk. I was crushed. I didn't know what to do. I didn't even know if my ankle would ever work again. The doctor's advice at the prison (after zero treatment) was: "Why do you play basketball? Don't do that. It's not good for you." When I asked for an ankle brace to support my ankle so that I could begin running on an unstable track again, I was told: "You don't need to run; you'll just hurt yourself. Your body doesn't need that . . ." What? So the medical advice I got was for no physical activity . . . ever. Apparently people don't need exercise for health. Where do they hire these people?

All that hard work for nothing. Thinking it was all over, I began to give up. Then inspiration hit! My brain, thankfully, kicked in as it had multiple times before when my body wouldn't cooperate with my inner drive. Through my constant reading (remember Chapter 2), I came across an article about *low-impact cardio*. I already knew about swimming, since this was something that I had long dreamed of returning to (there are no pools in prison), but I had never considered biking—not sure why, since there was one in the gym that I walked past every day before starting my workout. I also remember reading about a relatively new training method called High-Intensity Interval Training (HIIT), where I could basically hop on a bike and get more work done in less time than if I were jogging. I was back in action! Thank you, brain!!!

Here's how it works. HIITs are essentially short bursts of all-out energy expenditure followed by short periods of rest. Yes, you read that right. It's pure hell! By pushing your body harder than normal for these short periods of time and not letting it fully recover, you end up advancing your cardiovascular and musculature limits. The science behind all of this is very detailed of course, and I would suggest you read it for yourself, but all you need to know for now is that it works *damn well*. So well I can't believe you're not doing it right now. What are you waiting for!

In many ways this is also more beneficial than low-intensity, steady-state cardio where you essentially move at a steady, slower pace, for a prolonged period of time. A good example would be a person's typical jogging session. As noted above, you're not only expanding your cardiovascular capacity and building stronger, faster muscles, you're actually burning more calories in less time than dealing with those long, drawn-out jogs! Who wouldn't love that?

This form of cardio, which can be done in endless ways, also boosts your metabolism and leaves you burning more calories while you're doing anything, absolutely nothing at all, or even . . . watching TV! Amazing! See how lazy I really am? Between this and the Big Six Moves, I can watch TV all day and burn loads of unnecessary calories! TV's bad, though, don't watch it. Eats the mind.

This was the final piece of the puzzle. Just what I needed to achieve the body I desired and to attain impeccable health. It actually doesn't take too much cardio to maintain your looks and stay healthy once you get the ball rolling. Try a few varieties of HIITs on different apparatuses with varying time durations to see what works best for you. A good place to start would be with intervals of 15 seconds on and 45 seconds off. I recommend staying in the one-minute range so when that becomes manageable you can push yourself to 20 seconds on and 40 seconds off. Then try 25 seconds on and 35 seconds off . . . so on and so on. Here's a few examples of what I did in prison and what I still do to this day.

My favorite interval is on a stationary bike. I feel as though I get the most out of this particular exercise because it works my upper legs so intensely and in such a short period of time that I can barely manage to walk afterward. So what do I do? Once I'm warmed up, which I generally am after a good workout, I start my intervals. I simply do six sets taking only one minute each. That's it. A six-minute workout that will floor almost anyone you know and give you all types of benefits, from increased endurance to stronger muscles. Just use the method described earlier and do 20 seconds as hard as you can possibly go, followed by 40 seconds of walking or peddling to catch your breath, and repeat. That's it! To mix it up you could also do this on a rowing machine with moderate resistance or even a tread-mill with a slight incline, as I often find myself doing.

You get the point. And, contrary to popular belief, cardio doesn't have to be boring. Here's why . . .

Cardio: How Much Do I Really Need?

When it comes to cardio, people are often confused by how much they really need. It ultimately varies greatly for each person depending on your goals, where you're at physically, and, most important, how you feel. Basic recommendations for the average person would be 30 minutes of moderate exercise three times a week, but as far as I'm concerned, this is far too broad. To me this would be appropriate only for basic maintenance.

So how much do you really need? If you're not quite at the maintenance phase yet (where you've already attained the majority of your goals and now just want to keep up), I'd suggest training more frequently. In fact, I'd go as far as to engage in cardio exercise six days a week, especially if weight loss is your main goal. Re-member, you want to start off slowly so that your body has time to adapt to the additional strain. It's important not to push yourself too hard, or you'll likely end up setting yourself back.

Here's where working out smarter comes into play. If you're looking to burn fat fast, then focus on those dreaded HIITs. They work better and in less time than steady-state cardio, and this may soon become your new best friend. While I highly recommend performing HIITs two to three times a week, I'd also recom-mend getting in some steady-state cardio (when you simply set a pace and go, e.g., jogging, riding a bike, or swimming) as well, since it has a different set of benefits and won't push the body too hard. Both approaches are good and I've seen them work miracles for people. In my opinion, mixing the two is your best bet because your body won't know what to expect and you're less likely to overdo one or the other.

There are many ways to get your cardio fix, from swimming, biking, and rowing to stair climbers, box jumps, or just plain old jogging. Find what works best for you and stick to it. All of these activities can be performed at steady-state or at HIIT rates, so your options are limitless. Now you just have to find your plan and your stride. A quick example of how to use these exercises in both steady state and HIITs would be using the stair climber at a consistent, unchanged pace of say, level eight, for 30 minutes. This is steady-state cardio. If you wanted to take this same exercise to the next level, all you'd have to do is alternate difficulty settings on a stair climber from say a level five to a level 15 in one-minute cycles. So, try 15 seconds on level 15 going all out and then drop it to level five for a "rest" of 45 seconds. That's one cycle. Do this six to as many times as you can for a great HIIT workout. As stated earlier, it's just that simple!

Of course, sports have a role in all of this, too. If you play sports, this is an incredibly fun way to shed extra pounds. Personally, I'd recommend sports that really raise your activity level such as basketball, soccer, or even ultimate Frisbee. Put it this way, you're not going to burn too many calories bowling. But remember, any sport you play won't replace steady-state cardio or high-intensity interval training. Look at sports as more of a supplement, used to enhance your gains and of course to have some fun! The more active your lifestyle, the better off you'll be both mentally and physically, so get out there and play!

The Take

- Cardio is essential whether or not you're attempting to lose weight.
- Two to three days of cardio weekly are necessary for basic maintenance.
- Perform cardio six days a week with shorter workouts to lose weight.
- Cardio routines should involve steady-state training and HIIT. You can add various sports to supplement your program.
- Start out slow and build up your mileage and endurance. Your body needs time to adjust.
- Keep your cardio fresh by rotating different activities (swimming, biking, and jogging are just a few choices).

5

*The second day of a diet is always easier than the first.
By the second day you're off it.*

—JACKIE GLEASON

The Forever Diet

So you're working out, hitting the weights, and getting your cardio fix, yet you're still not in the shape you want to be. What gives?

Unfortunately, as most people discover when they try to create their best-possible physique, working out can only get you so far. Plain and simple, if you're not eating right, your progress will be severely limited. In fact, I would go so far as to say that a proper diet is the single most important component to developing the body of your dreams. You can spend all day in the gym, but if you're not feeding your muscles what they need to grow, they won't. Also, if you're eating too much fat or too many simple carbs, you'll end up undoing all that hard work on the weights or at the track. Mark my words, diet will transform you!

In my experience, far too many people overlook this crucial component, this daily consumption of energy that separates the ripped from the ranks. Like so much of the advice in this book, there's nothing especially fancy about a solid diet. Despite what you might read in various books and magazines, it's quite simple. There's no wonder drug or designer diet pill to act as a shortcut. A good diet is simplicity in itself, and once you see the results that come from combining a good workout and balanced diet, you'll never want to gorge on pizza, burgers, and ice cream again . . . okay, maybe I won't go that far, but you will come to see how harmful and useless these comfort foods can be.

Looking back, I've always been pretty fortunate when it came to my food intake. While my family wasn't too concerned with a "healthy diet"—or any aspect of healthy living for that matter—we just lucked into eating a relatively well-balanced diet. You see, my mom simply insisted on cooking. I think for her it was more of a monetary issue than anything else, but whatever the reason, the food I grew up on was great and my body appreciated it. Eating out costs big bucks and my mom wasn't going for that, especially when she knew she could whip up a better alternative right there in her own kitchen. That said, Mom's still not mastered an alternative to my beloved Dairy Queen Blizzards! Shame . . .

Things changed when I left home for college and my personal diet began to slip. Like many students at the ripe old age of 18, I alternated between Top Ramen and Burger King. By 19, though, I began to find a few healthy alternatives and was rapidly learning the hows and whats of enlightened eating habits. Things were beginning to come together for me. My body was on track for incredible growth and I was amazed at how it had aesthetically changed with just a base level of knowledge. Then my diet took a drastic turn for the worse. My arrest changed the way I would eat for the next 10 years, and not in a good way.

Cold, dank, county-jail food quickly became my one and only option as each day I was fed three of the most pathetic not-so-square meals that always left my stomach yearning for more and my taste buds reeling. Remember those lunches they served in the elementary school cafeteria? A little pasta, maybe some sauerkraut and a hot dog if you got lucky, that odd rectangle-shaped pizza that had no taste since it was 99 percent dough? Oh, how about those cute little cartons of milk or juice? Yep, that's what I was forced to eat as an adult, for more than a year and a half! Only difference was, back in school, I could get seconds. Never a full belly in the county. That should be their motto. It's an odd feeling to shudder at the taste of your food while at the same time wishing your captors would give you just a bit more to suppress your hunger pangs.

Fortunately, there was occasionally a bit of relief. For those lucky few who had the funds to afford it, one could purchase a couple boxes of Nutty Bars and maybe even a few Dunkin' Sticks each week. This was hardly enough to fill the void, but if timed correctly, these "treats" could at least quiet the growl in that empty pit of your stomach for a time.

For nearly two years this is how my life played out. While I waited for my eventual trial, my life was defined by the tedious battle to scrounge up enough food to try to get from one day to the next. This was my new reality. Who knew that county jail, where you're meant to be considered "innocent until proven guilty," would easily turn out to be the most oppressive, life-draining environment I would endure during my hellish 10 years in the Missouri justice system. No choices, no options, no nothing. No wonder I ate like a pig once I landed in prison.

I'll never forget the first opportunity I had to buy real food in nearly two years, after I left county jail and entered the prison system. To actually feel full was a frightening thought. I didn't know how to act. It felt like Christmas and, it being December 10, I guess it kind of was. I arrived at the prison diagnostic center on a snowy Tuesday night with not one cent and was told that the canteen would be open on Thursday morning (you go only once a week). If I missed this window of opportunity, it would mean more of the starving and suffering of the last two years, except this time, everyone around me would be getting full-on the delicious goodies they were able to buy at this very different facility. Luckily, someone let me use their phone time to call my go-to guy (my dad). He understood that it was almost impossible to get cash to the prison that quickly, but, in true Bill Ferguson spirit, confidently wired the money immediately. Of all the amazing things my dad's done for me, most of which are 100 times more important than this simple deed, I'll never forget his quick response.

Thirty-six hours later and it was my housing unit's turn to take a trip to the canteen. Coincidentally, and unbeknownst to me, the team from CBS's *48 Hours* had showed up at that same time. I was mortified. I needed food and wasn't at all ready for Erin Moriarty and her crew to film me for what could be my only chance to speak publicly for myself. I hadn't even had the opportunity to buy a razor to shave with. I looked like a sleep-deprived, half-starved wild bum. Not good!

Thankfully, it all came together. My celly gave me a razor. The guard gave me exactly five minutes to shave and shower, where I promptly cut my lip wide open, and I was on my way. It was then that I was told I could go to the canteen after my interview, while also being informed that as of 8:00 a.m. that morning I had about as much money as I came into this world with. I already knew I would be facing a long wait in prison while the courts sifted through the lies of the state and its agents, but this was not the start I was hoping for.

After an abbreviated interview through two thick inches of glass, which, although awkward, seemed to go pretty well in spite of the barrier, my immediate stress was over and it was back to my newfound hell of being a have-not surrounded by haves. As I moseyed back to my unit, enjoying the cool, crisp winter air I hadn't felt in two years while in county lockup, a thought occurred to me as we passed the canteen and I begged the CO to check my account one last time. The CO grudgingly obliged. We arrived at the machine, and after a seemingly endless wait while the screen updated, my account popped up: 200 dollars! YAHTZEE!

After happily standing outside for nearly an hour in the most refreshing winter weather I'd ever felt, I was able to purchase a hat, gloves, new shoes, and, even better, doughnuts, coffee, cigs, soups, and a summer sausage. Things I hadn't seen in more than a year and a half. Needless to say, I ate like a fiend, smoked, and drank coffee for three days straight. To hell with health. I had a choice!

For the next couple of years that's how I ate. To make matters worse, I accelerated this unhealthy diet in the misguided hope that, coupled with rigorous workouts, I might become large enough to scare away potential predators. Fortunately, as time went on, my continued reading and education taught me the error of my ways, and I soon realized I would have to get my diet back on track.

Turns out, diets are somewhat confounding to a person first attempting to figure it all out. The most important lesson I learned was the devastating realization that most people are unhealthy not because they consciously choose to eat terrible food, but because of widespread confusion.

As my thinking began to shift and I chose to move away from being as big and bad as possible to being as big and lean as possible, everything regarding my diet changed. I quickly realized that in order to maintain mass, while at the same time attempting to get lean, I had to reeducate myself and get health conscious. It's easy to simply get big (eat a lot and lift heavy), and it's easy to get lean (starve yourself and do lots of cardio), but doing both at the same time is a precise science that can take years to master on your own. (That is, of course, unless you have this book!)

Not knowing where to start, I began by learning about the nutritional labels on the back of typical everyday products. At the time, I knew nothing about food labeling. It all seemed totally foreign to me. What was the significance of all those fats, carbs, and calories, and what did all these numbers mean? More to the point, how much of each did I need in my diet?

The more I read, the more I learned and my whole diet quickly shifted. There are various ways to figure out how many calories each individual needs and how they should split these calories between fats, carbs, and proteins, which essentially constitute our diets (a.k.a. macronutrients). But the options can overwhelm and confuse people. That's why we'll skip most of the technical math and stick to basic nutritional guidelines: approximately 2,500 calories for men and 2,000 for women. This is what I worked with for years, and I couldn't have been happier with the results. When attempting to gain lean muscle (which is almost always), I consume 50 percent carbs, 30 percent protein, and 20 percent fat. Another division I use when I tailor back my workouts and want to indulge a bit is 45 percent carbs, 30 percent protein, and 25 percent fat. That said, it's best to experiment with different ratios and see what works best for your body.

One quick note! When doing these calculations, one must understand that there are 4 calories in one gram of carbs, 4 calories in one gram of protein, and a whopping 9 calories in one gram of fat. Here's an example of how you can calculate your ideal ratios in a 50/30/20 split based on a 2,500-calorie daily diet. Remember, this is similar to what a man of average size would use. Calculations for the average female would likely begin around 1,800 to 2,000 calories.

50% Carbs: 2,500 calories daily x .50 (percentage of carbs in your daily diet) = 1,250
1,250 calories of carbs daily ÷ 4 (calories in 1 gram of carbs) = 312.5
So . . . you'd need 312.5 grams of carbs per day.

30% Proteins: 2,500 calories daily x .30 (percentage of proteins in your daily diet) = 750
750 calories of proteins daily ÷ 4 (calories in 1 gram of protein) = 187.5
So . . . you'd need 187.5 grams of protein per day.

20% Fats: 2,500 calories daily x .20 (percentage of fats in your daily diet) = 500
500 calories of fats daily ÷ 9 (calories in 1 gram of fat) = 55.5
So . . . you'd need 55.5 grams of fat per day.

Daily intake: 312.5 grams of carbs/187.5 grams of protein/55.5 grams of fats

That's it. You don't have to be obsessive about these numbers of course, I'm certainly not, but the closer you are, the better off you'll be. If you want to lose weight, you can go into what's called a calorie deficit and safely drop between 200 and 500 calories per day. One pound of fat = 3,500 calories. So, the theory is, if you cut 500 calories per day for one week, it'll add up to 3,500 calories or one pound of weight. Just do the same calculations as above but start from 2,000 calories instead of 2,500 calories. It won't all be fat you lose, but it'll get you moving in the right direction. You just want to be sure to eat healthy, maintain your lean muscle mass, and go into deficits only every so often for a month or so. I've done it, but I shrank up, so I don't really like it. Only way to find out if it's for you is to try it.

What I do greatly enjoy is the calorie surplus. This is done when attempting to gain lean muscle mass. I increase my calories by about 200 per day while working out superhard, and it feels great. Note: if you exercise a lot, you may want to eat additional calories anyway. I do about 100 to 200 calories per hour I work out just because my body will burn off these calories, and without accounting for these burned calories, I'll place myself in a calorie deficit, thus hurting my gains. The same will apply for you.

As I slowly became aware of what my specific body type needed, and, more important, what it didn't, I went from daily burritos and beef stew meals topped with cheese, ranch dressing, chips, summer sausage, and beef tips to a standard meal of Top Ramen, refried beans, chicken or tuna, and jalapeños for added flavor. Keep in mind, my options in prison were pretty slim, but this one simple change immediately cut around 2,100 calories from my weekly diet (not to mention lots of unnecessary fats, carbs, and an extreme excess of sodium). I dropped 2,100 calories by changing just one daily meal over the course of one week! That was over a half pound of unnecessary garbage holding me back on a weekly basis. Over a year, that added up to more than 31 pounds of excess weight I would have had to work off. I didn't even want to begin thinking about how many miles I'd have to run to compensate for that amount of empty calories. My journey had begun!

After about a year of changing my eating habits and achieving some pretty fantastic results, I stumbled across my next big lesson, which we touched on in the preceding paragraph: the power of accumulation! One of the most common ways we sabotage our dreams of a better body is the intake of relatively small, seemingly harmless amounts of fats and sugars and other simple carbs eaten on a daily basis. While the quantities may seem insignificant in a single serving, a little sugar in your coffee or a dash of ranch on that healthy salad eventually adds up, and over the course of weeks and years, those small indulgences soon turn into those difficult bulges and bellies we just can't seem to get rid of.

Take that cup of coffee for example. Drinking it black adds up to around 10 or so calories, not so bad right? Then add just three small sugar cubes to spruce it up a little and you're good to go. No harm no foul, how terrible could those little cubes be? Well . . . that little change adds 12 grams of sugar, 12 grams of carbs, and 45 calories. That's still a better option than your average soda, but 45 totally unnecessary calories? It may not sound like much, but let's do the math over the course of a month. That's 1,350 useless calories! That's almost a whole day's worth of calories for a typical female and more than half for a typical male. How about over a whole year? It's 16,425 calories and 4,380 grams of sugar. That's almost 10 pounds of sugar and more than 10 days' worth of calories for a female! That's just ONE example of ONE cup of coffee, with no creamer or additional additives.

Now, how much easier do you think it would be to meet your goals if you didn't have to work off nearly 10 pounds of sugar and 10 extra days' worth of food each year? How much less work would you have to do in the gym? Life altering!

Small Changes = Big Results

So maybe you don't drink coffee. How about the fatty dressings you use on your salad or the way you cook your food? While butter and cooking oil may be better for you than most cooking sprays, how much of it do you use? It might not seem like much, but it adds up. What alternatives are out there? Coconut oil is my go-to since it has healthy fats, but there are other options out there for you to research and experiment with that may fit your calorie and taste needs. While we're on the subject, don't be tricked into the "light" or "low-fat" versions of these condiments . . . check the sugars, fats, carbs, and ingredients. The label tells the story.

With this fundamental understanding about nutrition now paying dividends both mentally and physically, I was gradually developing a body beyond my dreams. The results were amazing, and I hadn't even changed that much in my life. Feeling good about myself, I could have stayed on course and felt great, but I knew there was more to be learned and about seven years into my journey toward the goal of perfect health and fitness the easy way, I stumbled upon my greatest discovery yet.

If Man Made It, Don't Eat It!

Simple fact: most processed foods are terrible for us. Come on, you've seen the labels with the impossible-to-pronounce ingredients, the preservatives, additives, and Frankenfoods, which clearly don't exist in nature! Now I'll admit, cutting processed foods out of your diet IS more of a lifestyle change than the other suggestions I've offered so far, but in my experience, it wasn't anywhere near as difficult to make as I first thought it might be. It's as simple as learning the staples of your diet and staying away from pretty much every aisle on the inside of the supermarket. Do this and you'll be good to go. Why would you want to eat a salad dressing that has 30 ingredients on the label? How "natural" can that be? It can't. Why? Because it's not. Vinegar and extra-virgin olive oil are a great alternative. Two ingredients, a wonderful taste, and few calories. I love it! Plus you get some healthy essential fats out of one!

As I switched over to my new, healthier diet, two key factors were at the forefront of my mind: (1) having enough flavor and variety to keep my diet interesting; and (2) maintaining an ample supply of lean protein. At first I thought this would prove difficult, but thankfully, over time, it became less and less of a challenge.

The short and skinny of this plan is to aim for a plant-based diet with plenty of fruits and vegetables; lean meats such as chicken and fish for protein; and good, whole grains for additional complex carbs, found in quinoa and Ezekiel bread, for example, to give you sustained energy. This diet includes plenty of other foods to get you through the day—such as eggs, yogurt, oatmeal, nuts, and lean beef jerky—but be careful when it comes to snacking since the calories add up fast! If you eat these foods consistently and work out regularly, you'll likely find it difficult NOT to slim down and muscle up. Remember, this is *your* diet, not *a* diet. You're embarking on a new *life*style.

By ridding yourself of all those harmful chemicals and additives, studies show that you may live longer and you'll enjoy a better quality of life. Plus, you'll likely end up eating fewer calories on a daily basis, since unadulterated foods are generally less calorie dense and are full of good, healthy carbs, which help keep you fuller longer. So once again, what are you waiting for?

Portion Control

Changing my own diet in prison had a profound effect on my body and truly separated me from the herd. In less than a year, I was more shredded and had built so much more mass that even the biggest bad asses began asking for pointers. Best of all, I wasn't working any harder than before. I just switched up my diet and stayed consistent. It was that easy. And then, just when I thought I'd figured out my whole diet, the final two pieces of the puzzle fell into place: portion size and meal timing.

We begin with portion sizes. Let's be real, portion sizes in America are out of control. Even Benjamin Franklin knew this more than two hundred years ago, saying, "To lengthen thy life, lessen thy meals." But somewhere along the way we as a nation forgot this. Studies show that most Americans have no idea what an appropriate portion of food looks like, and the problem is only getting worse.

Our diets are deteriorating on a daily basis, not only because of what companies put in their food, but because of how much *we* put on our plate. On average, the serving you receive at any major restaurant is two to four times larger than necessary. Think of all those extra calories. The excess fats and carbs have nowhere to go but our guts and our butts. Even if restaurants served healthy food this would still be a bad situation. Two-thirds of the U.S. population is now overweight or obese. It's no wonder we can't keep up in the gym. We've been inadvertently undermining our efforts for years. Is it any surprise that so many people struggle to lose weight "no matter what they try"?

Measure your food. If you're making the healthiest meals at home, but eating huge portions, you're still going nowhere fast. Keep it simple. The recommended serving size of meat per meal is three ounces, or the size of a deck of cards. Do you like snacking on healthy almonds, walnuts, or dried fruits? Great! Measure out a fourth of a cup per day and put the bag away. That's about one ounce or the size of a golf ball. You should stick to around one cup of berries and vegetables per meal, which is about the size of a baseball. Don't overindulge at all, stick to what's good for you, and you'll see results. You'll also become aware of how much you used to eat. And here's an interesting fact that I find most enjoyable: food = money, so think about that added benefit as well. Less food = more discretionary cash!

Here's some more good news. Just as our stomachs grow to meet the demands of an excessive diet, they will shrink once portion control begins. As I began eating smaller and smaller portions of healthy food, my body responded over time, and pretty soon I stopped craving excess calories. All it takes is awareness and a little patience. Think of it this way, would you rather work off the amount of food you just ate, enough to feed two people, or would you prefer to save yourself the trouble and not put all those unnecessary calories in your mouth to begin with? For me, the answer was easy; it just took a little getting used to.

Imagine this: it takes only 15 minutes to consume a 1,200-calorie meal (an incredibly easy affair at many restaurants these days), but it would take you two long hours of running at five miles per hour just to burn off those same calories. That being said, you'd have to exercise eight times longer than it took to eat that meal in the first place, and you'd have to put in an exorbitant quantity of work to even things back up. Sound like fun? No, thank you! Remember that one pound of fat equals 3,500 calories. There's a good chance that you're consuming an additional 1,000 calories beyond your needs each day (and that's a conservative estimate). Every four days you're adding ONE WHOLE POUND of unnecessary garbage to your frame. WOW! Think about that! And you thought that sugar-laden coffee was bad.

When to Eat

Last, but certainly not least, we come to the science of timing our food intake. Studies vary a fair bit on this topic. But, when it comes to the two most important meals of the day, your breakfast and postworkout meals, you won't find a whole lot of debate. A healthy, well-balanced breakfast with about 20 to 40 grams of protein; some simple carbs in the form of fructose (think an apple, banana, orange, or blueberries, to name a few choices); and about 30 to 70 grams of complex carbs, depending on whether you're attempting to gain or lose weight. Think oats, whole grains, all-bran cereal, shredded wheat, spinach, kale . . . the list goes on. This should offer a good start to your day, and it will kick-start your metabolism, help regulate your blood-sugar levels, and fight against hunger throughout the day. All this while also boosting your energy levels! So . . . EAT BREAKFAST. Oh, I hate to be the bearer of bad news, but your Tootie Fruities and doughnuts don't count. That stuff is pure junk and will start your day in a deficit. Not a breakfast person? Make a shake. Throw in a scoop of protein powder or Greek yogurt, fruit of your choice, spinach, flaxseed, and voilà! Drink down your breakfast, then a few hours later, grab something a bit more substantial. This is generally what I do. There are no excuses!

Your postworkout meal is also incredibly important. After exercising, there's an approximately 30-minute window when your muscles are primed for their maximum uptake of macronutrients such as protein and carbs. So it's best to utilize this window in order to make the most of your workouts. This is imperative if you're looking to build lean muscle and create a healthy lifestyle. Look at it this way, if you don't take the opportunity to use this window, you'll be wasting a significant portion of your workouts.

Studies have shown that a postworkout shake of whey protein powder and casein protein powder are superior to whey alone. These supplements are better than whole foods because they can be absorbed faster (whey) or slower (casein), so that your body gets the nutrients it desires in the appropriate frame of time. That's why I drink a shake of 25 grams of whey and 25 grams of casein immediately after working out. About an hour to an hour and a half later, I make myself a whole foods meal with about 70 grams of carbs and 30 grams of protein to ensure balanced eating habits and to stay in an anabolic (building muscle) state. As you can see, supplements are important. We will talk about supplements more in the following chapter.

There are a few other important food-schedule slots, but before we get too far along I'd like to venture back to that all-important breakfast. If you choose to do cardio in the morning and would like to burn a little extra fat, then this is the only reason you can have for skipping breakfast. This is a hotly debated subject, but certain studies show that doing so makes your body pull energy from fat reserves, and this is obviously a good thing if you're looking to get lean as quickly as possible. If you choose to do cardio at this time, you should hydrate and consider taking branched-chain amino acids (BCAAs). These are used to stimulate the building of protein in muscle, which can improve exercise performance in athletes and reduce muscle breakdown. BCAAs combined with good hydration is my game plan before every morning workout, now that I have that option. Once your cardio session is done, it's supplement time. The whey-and-casein mix we spoke of earlier, along with a piece of fruit for carbs, would be perfect immediately after this a.m. exercise. An hour and a half later, try to eat about 30 to 50 grams of both proteins and carbs, respectively. This number should be sufficiently filling and will provide you with the nutrients to recover as well as be enough to give you ample supplies of energy for your morning. Remember: this is the ONLY reason you should have for skipping breakfast. Don't abuse it, it'll only hurt your waistline.

From here we'll skip all the way to the other end of the day, late night. Conventional wisdom would have us believe that you should endeavor not to eat within a two-hour window before bedtime or you'll end up like the fat guy on that Austin Powers movie. Well, all I gotta say is, screw conventional wisdom. It's flat-out wrong. All that matters at this particular WHEN is WHAT you eat. Sure, fatty foods and simple carbs will inevitably turn into lard. This means nothing, though. We already know that, right? The reality is that these foods will do so at the same rate any time of day. If fact, they may be even worse for you in the morning since they'll lead to a crash while zapping your energy supplies, thus leaving you as nothing more than a useless ball of lazy. Ever felt that way? I sure have. Next time it happens, think about what you ate that morning.

In opposition to the "never eat before bedders," I say go right ahead and eat up. I do it every night and my abs seem to love it. All you have to do is . . . eat healthy. Revolutionary, huh? Low-fat milk and cereal are a good, proven nighttime snack. The mix of complex carbs from the cereal and protein from the milk ensure that you'll be headed into slumber with an adequate supply of nutrients to feed an active body. Casein protein (slow digesting so that nutrients trickle through your body as you sleep) is also a good choice for those looking to develop lean muscle. Consuming casein prior to bed ensures that your body will stay in an anabolic state (growing muscle) instead of entering a fasting state where there will be no nutrients to feed the demands of a well-exercised body. It's common sense, really. Muscles, being made of protein, need protein to grow. Just don't feed them too much and they'll use it all up as you rest. I stick to a casein with as few ingredients as possible and stay away from vegan proteins, which generally cost more and don't absorb as well. That, however, is a personal choice all must make.

In between these two main feeding times and your workouts, your meal timing can be a little less strict. Just try to get 20 to 40 grams of protein and 30 to 70 grams of carbs in your body every two or three hours or so and you'll be good to go. Studies also vary here but this timing theoretically helps keep your muscles in an anabolic state throughout the day while also giving you sustained energy. More than that and you'll be overdoing it. What's more important here is eating enough to provide energy while splitting your calories into manageable portions throughout the day. Although nutrients are digested at wildly different rates, it's still good to spread them out and simply make sure that you reach your daily caloric goals. You can drive yourself crazy with studies on how often to eat, so just keep your eyes on the big picture. Once you've used up all these nutrients, your muscles become hungry again, and, as we all know, you've gotta feed the beast.

I call this way of eating the "Forever Diet" because it's a *lifestyle,* NOT a diet. One thing all my research and experience have taught me is that no arbitrary short-term "diet" is going to give you the long-term benefits of remaining consistently lean and muscular. Eventually the yo-yo effect will take over and the unsustainability of fad dieting will hurt you in the long term. When this happens, and it will happen, you'll likely find your body shape as well as your weight in perpetual fluctuation. How demoralizing is that?

This is why I don't believe in "diets." As long as you create and consistently adhere to a healthy, well-balanced lifestyle, you should never need to go on another "diet." Now, you can, and should, have a few cheat meals; but the days of crazy eating should be gone for good. Trying to stick to an unrealistic diet is simply setting yourself up for failure.

Keep It Casual

As you've undoubtedly realized by now, I'm not a huge fan of a strictly regimented lifestyle. Although there is a time and a place for being tightly disciplined, that's not what this book is about. My goal is to achieve the look of someone who is intensely regimented without deviating so far from an ordinary lifestyle that it becomes no longer fun or sustainable. That's why I recommend dedicating yourself to lots of small, functional, and hopefully manageable changes that fit into a BALANCED lifestyle.

I suggest using an approach similar to the workout structure I've outlined, whereby you alternate your GO-TO "main" meals with a group of more INTERCHANGEABLE "secondary" meals. The first should be your perfect, nutritionally sound basics that you love and can fit into your lifestyle with ease. The second would be your substitute meals, perhaps a little less sound but still generally healthy, and your snacks. Below are just a few examples of my daily intake. As you can see, there are several options in each category. These are just general examples; you can replace any meat, fruit, or veggie with your favorites. Try them out, mix them up, and create your own meal plans! Keep in mind, portion sizes are going to be different for everyone because everyone has different intake needs and goals. Calculate the portion sizes to accommodate your personal requirements.

Go-To Food Options	
Breakfast	• 2 eggs, Ezekiel-bread toast, 1 cup blueberries • ½ cup plain Greek yogurt with 1 cup mixed fruit • 1 cup cooked oatmeal with 1 banana and ½ cup blueberries • green smoothie (1 cup of spinach and kale, half an apple, 1 cup pineapple, ½ cup water, 2 celery stalks) • protein shake
Lunch	• tuna salad (4 oz. canned tuna packed in water; ½ cup Greek yogurt; 1 celery stalk, chopped fine; 1 hard-boiled egg, mashed; ½ small avocado; ½ cup spinach); ½ piece whole-grain pita bread; 1 cup fruit; tomato-and-cucumber salad topped with oil and vinegar • 4 ounces of broiled/grilled/baked chicken, shredded and served on top of a spinach salad with ½ cup strawberries, oil and vinegar
Dinner	• 4 ounces broiled/grilled/baked salmon, 1 cup veggies, ½ cup quinoa or brown rice, ½ cup cottage cheese • 4 oz. grilled chicken, salad (1 cup spinach, 1/3 cup chopped tomato, ½ cup cucumber, 2 oz. oil/2 oz. vinegar dressing, 1 medium-sized sweet potato)
Snacks	• 1 cup fruit • 1 cup veggies • hard-boiled egg • protein shake • green smoothie • nuts • dark chocolate

Interchangeables	
Breakfast	• egg, tomato, and ½ avocado on a whole wheat English muffin • 2 pieces Ezekiel toast, 2 tablespoons peanut butter, sliced banana
Lunch	• grilled chicken wrap, 1 cup grapes, ⅓ cup mixed nuts
Dinner	• 4 ounces of steak, baked or grilled • sweet potato, baked • vegetable medley
Snacks	• rice cake with 2 tablespoons peanut butter • 1 cup popped plain popcorn • hummus • kale chips • pretzels • ⅓ cup guacamole with carrots and celery • pistachios • Ezekiel toast with peanut butter and a sliced banana • 2 tablespoons raisins

As you can see, it all comes down to planning. If you take the time up front to create a list of healthy, portion-appropriate, well-timed meals and pair these with proper hydration, your daily food choices will become little more than a matter of filling in the empty spaces of a chart. Point, click, and you're done. It's just that easy. As long as you stick to this casual plan 95 percent of the time and don't deviate too far from the whats, whens, and hows of this diet, your body will have almost no other option than to burn fat and build muscle, and you can keep eating this way FOREVER!

To simplify things even more, I generally cook a couple cups of steel-cut oats, five chicken breasts, and a few cups of quinoa at the beginning of each week so all I have to do is pull it out, microwave it for a few, add a salad or some eggs, and voilà! I'm happily fed and healthy. There are all types of similar shortcuts and quick fixes to make life easier. I enjoy hunting for new ways to save time and energy and improve my health all at once. It's all about the continuation of education!

What to Drink

Food is, of course, crucially important, but let's not forget the dynamic role of proper hydration. If you drink badly—think soda, excessive alcohol, sugary fruit juices, and so on—you can quickly undo all your dietary work.

If I asked you to tell me the difference between a 160-calorie cupcake with 40 grams of sugar and your typical soda, what would your answer be? As far as calories, sugars, and carbs go, there isn't a whole lot of difference, but how much more likely are you to reject the cupcake, thinking you're doing something good for yourself, while consuming the sugary beverage? We've all done it; to make matters worse, high-calorie drinks do not fill you up, so chances are you'll end up eating excess calories either with or after that sugary soda!

As bad as soda is, it's not the only dietary danger. Juices, energy drinks, coffee, alcohol, and pretty much any beverage besides water can have this same destructive effect. They all contain calories, which will either take the place of more nutritious, more filling options or will just be added to the food you're already putting in your body. If you think the accumulation from a few sugar cubes was bad, try adding up just one sugary beverage daily over the course of a month or a year and figure out how many miles you'd have to run to burn those babies off! So drink carefully!

By now I hope I've sold you on the benefits of water. If not, here are a few more! First, water is the ultimate source of hydration. A lack of proper hydration leaves us with less energy to tackle each day and can cause numerous physical issues such as skin problems, migraines, depression, and even constipation, to name just a few. Studies have shown that over half of us are chronically dehydrated, and I believe it. Conventional wisdom says that we should drink about eight eight-ounce glasses of water a day, and while this isn't an exact calculation, it's likely a lot more than most people are currently drinking. A better estimation of how much we should consume on a daily basis is:

Your body weight × 0.5 + 12 × number of hours exercised = Ounces of water per day.

For example: I weigh 170 pounds, so I'd take . . . 170 × 0.5 = 85

And I work out about an hour each day, so that's 12 × 1 = 12

Then you add these totals up: 85 + 12 = 97 fluid ounces of water per day. (So I need to drink about 12 × 8-ounce glasses of water per day, or 5 of the 20-ounce cups I keep around.)

Given all the benefits it provides, why don't more people drink more water? My guess is because it's difficult for most of us to keep track of everything we consume, and in the midst of our busy lives, we forget the basics. Once again, you must PLAN!

As you can see, I drink about 100 fluid ounces of water a day. To make this goal manageable, I make sure to drink whole 20-ounce cups at key times of the day and simply sip from my cup at others. For example, I drink one whole 20-ounce cup when I wake up, another two hours prior to working out, one immediately after working out, and one about an hour before dinner. That leaves me with one unaccounted-for cup, which I sip throughout the day. It's just that easy. So no excuses, start drinking your daily water.

The Take

- There are no such things as "diets," this is a LIFESTYLE.
- Proper dieting habits can make or break the possibility of reaching your goals regardless of how much you work out.
- Avoid eating out.
- Stick to a mostly plant-based diet with lean meats for adequate protein.
- Not all processed food is bad, just 99 percent of it. Avoid man-made food when you can.
- You can count calories without being obsessive about it. It just takes a little investment in time up front.
- Plan your go-to and interchangeable meals of small amounts of fats or calories.
- Be wary of accumulation!
- Your diet can be both healthy and interesting.
- Be sure to hit the important eating windows: breakfast, preworkout, postworkout, and before bed. Outside of this, spread out your meals so they're manageable to consume.
- To make life easier, mass cook whatever you can at the beginning of the week.
- Stay hydrated!

6

Sell yourself short on nutrition and you're selling
yourself short on maximizing your physical development.

—ERNIE TAYLOR

Maximizing Your Gains: Rest, Recovery, and Supplements

Overwhelming. If this is how you feel when facing the daunting world of supplements, you aren't alone. Outside of bodybuilders, personal trainers, and nutritionists (who often seem to contradict each other), no one seems to quite know what works and what doesn't in this billion-dollar industry.

Adding to the confusion is the multitude of infomercials, bad websites, and copycat magazines that are little more than glorified advertising vehicles for endorsements. So what are we to make of all these claims? If these products work, why isn't everyone on them? Where should you even start?

It's simple actually, so simple it only took me a few years to sort through all the varying theories and research to come up with the approach that I'm about to share with you. And this is just the beginning. I'm sure my research into this field will last a lifetime, but like everything else in this book, it can be summarized in four words . . . STICK TO THE BASICS.

First off, I believe it's important to understand that supplements are just that: supplements. They are not there to replace the foods we eat, which should come primarily from the all-natural, minimally processed sources we discussed in the previous chapter. Instead, supplements exist to give us that extra little nutritional boost that nature, in its current state, can't always fulfill.

That's why it's important to understand *why* we choose to supplement. Before we go in depth about which supplements to use, we need to understand their place in the world of fitness. While there are many forms and uses for supps, we'll stick to what I believe we need them for most: a phase of our development referred to as "rest and recovery." So without further ado, let's look at that all-important *why* of supplementation starting with that all-important rest part of our rest and recovery.

You see, when you're in prison, you lack many essential nutrients and suffer from a severe lack of protein (no bodybuilding.com inside I'm afraid). But there is one key workout requirement that you have in abundance. Rest.

Like it or not, the chances are quite high that finding adequate rest won't be a major problem when you're locked down 21 to 24 hours a day. It's exceedingly difficult to expend a great deal of energy in prison. This is especially true when a majority of that time is spent with some random psychopathic celly. There are exceptions, naturally, like this crazy guy in ad-seg (a.k.a. "the hole"), who supposedly performed 5,000 sit-ups a day. That is, until he "broke" his abs. Strained, tore, or severely injured them is likely what happened, but "broke" just sounds better.

Since rest periods in prison were unavoidable, I often found myself sleeping up to 15 hours a day. I spent many of my waking hours reading, playing chess, or catching up on the news, and, of course, working out. But even exercise proved challenging at times. When you live in an oppressive cage devoid of sunlight, nutrition, or even an adequate supply of clean clothes, it can be hard to scrounge up the necessary motivation to hit the weights.

Nonetheless, as my workouts progressed, along with my exercise education, so did my understanding of the human body. I already knew the long-standing bodybuilding principle of not working the same muscle group two days in a row, but I didn't know why. Eventually I learned that this 48-hour principle was actually part of the much larger scientific understanding mentioned earlier: "rest and recovery" (or R&R for short), a whole field of knowledge that includes the use of supplements, the need for adequate sleep, and an index of multiple training methods. Used correctly, these principles can save you a lot of time, effort, and energy. Who wouldn't want these kinds of shortcuts?

That's why the art of R&R is, without a doubt, my favorite requirement when it comes to getting fit and healthy. It also happens to be something I'm rather good at! After all, who doesn't love the principle of chugging a giant strawberry-banana shake (more on this later) and sleeping it off?

Hold on, though, not so fast! While you may be thinking of how enjoyable this all sounds, let me sound a note of caution. This chapter is all about getting the RIGHT kind of rest, recovery, and supplements. Yep, even here there is work involved! Getting into great shape isn't just about working hard at the gym and sleeping the rest of the day. Here's what you need to know.

The first thing one must understand is that muscles do not "grow" in the gym. Contrary to popular belief, they actually grow while in the process of recovery (postworkout). Numerous studies explain this whole physiological miracle in detail. However, in a nutshell, what they're all basically saying is this: the more weight you use, the greater the amount of muscle fibers you'll be breaking down. This means that when you work out at the gym lifting weights, running, or pushing your aerobic capacity, you're actually tearing apart microscopic muscle fibers and wreaking havoc on your body (yep, that's why those squats hurt so darn much!).

Once you leave the gym, your body then begins repairing these muscle fibers, thus bringing them back bigger and stronger so that they can continue to fight future stresses. It's evolution at its best! If you allow your muscles to heal properly, which takes about a minimum of 48 hours, and supplement with protein, which is what muscle is composed of, then, voilà! Your muscles will start to grow.

Supplement with protein? Yes, protein is essential to your muscle growth. Since your muscles are composed primarily of water and protein, it is good to get adequate amounts of both to your muscles as quickly as possible. I touched on this in the previous chapter, and I'll speak fully about it later in this chapter. For now, let's remember that there is a short window, approximately 30 minutes postworkout, where your body is primed to absorb more nutrients to help aid in the process of repairing torn muscle fibers. Studies have shown that people who take advantage of this window, supplementing with quick-digesting whey protein, experience better lean-muscle gains while also reducing soreness. There's a double benefit; you'll be back in the gym working that same area of the body sooner and with more muscle than if you had ignored this portion of your recovery.

Hand in hand with recovery and getting the proper nutrients in your body postworkout is then *resting* whatever muscles you exerted. The definition of rest is very subjective and can easily be taken out of context. Knowing how this terminology is used in the world of health and fitness may vary a bit from what you're accustomed to hearing, so let me clarify. Resting muscle groups essentially means not working out the same part of the body two days in a row, even longer in some cases. The process of repairing your muscle fibers takes approximately this long, so working out sooner could lead to injury and diminish your gains.

Another form of rest is a good night's sleep. Naps may be helpful as well, but not so much that we should spend our time talking about them here. Their benefits simply aren't on a scale large enough to actively incorporate into most training regimens. Suffice to say, you cannot make up for a lack of sleep with naps. *Shoot for eight hours!* Next to an active lifestyle and healthy diet, the need for sleep is undoubtedly the most important factor when it comes to achieving and maintaining optimum health. During the course of the day we use up a multitude of chemicals that occur naturally in our body, which will never replenish if we don't get enough shut-eye. Without the proper levels of these chemicals in our bodies, our minds and our muscles will eventually become inefficient and stymie our progress, and trust me, you don't even want to know about the long-term effects of a lack of sleep. For most of us, this means about six to nine hours per night. I need about nine, but from what I can see, I'm just strange. So eat right, take your supplements, train smart, and SLEEP!

So as you can see . . . YOU MUST REST! If you don't allow your muscles to fully recover, not only do your results suffer down the line but your risk of injury increases immensely.

Similar to what we talked about in the previous chapter: Small Changes = Big Results. Like many great things in life, it all adds up over time. Your body will thank you! With the whys of rest and recovery now understood, we can venture into the land of supplementation. Unfortunately, this is not nearly as simple as sleeping and taking days off. By the end of this chapter, though, you will be on your way to supplementing your R&R properly. What's even better is that you can avoid following the slightly tragic, slightly humorous journey I took to get this knowledge!

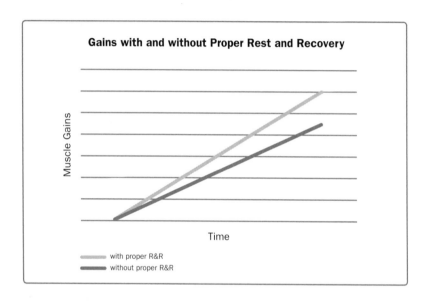

The Roast Beef Regimen

My first foray into the world of supplementation was in 2006. After being formally introduced to penitentiary workouts, I soon realized that if my efforts were breaking my muscles down, something—protein—was essential in building them back up.

Armed with this most basic concept of postworkout recovery, yet lacking any proper supplements, I embarked on a journey to find my own protein source. At this stage, I assumed that all protein was created equal, so my plan was simple: find whatever product the canteen sold that possessed the highest amount of protein, for the best price, and eat as much as possible after working out.

That is how my roast beef regimen began. Beef WAS available in prison, and while it was somewhat high in fat, it had the protein necessary for two postworkout meals, while having the added benefit of tasting good. It was also a good excuse to spend money on something that I would otherwise have considered a luxury.

The best part . . . it worked. After about two years of this meat (and fat) assault on my body, I packed on some serious muscle.

The Milk Affair

It was about this time that I started to learn a new lesson. All protein, it turns out, is NOT created equal, and the rate at which these different proteins are absorbed by your body can make a huge difference in your gains. I realized that I wasn't getting enough protein from beef immediately after my workouts.

Meat, it turns out, takes too long to absorb to be highly effective during that critical 30 minutes postworkout, when your body is primed to soak up the higher amounts of nutrition it needs for growth and recuperation. On top of that, there is the fat issue! Unknown by me at the time, I was taking in way too much fat, even though I was highly active. Therefore, no matter how hard I tried, I could never reach my ultimate goal: achieving a lean, athletic look.

That is when my love affair with milk began! After years of believing I had to put up with copious amounts of fat to obtain a proper level of protein, I came across an article for endurance athletes that provided a breakthrough. I realized *I could grow muscle without adding fat*. I know it may sound crazy, but the theory has good evidence backing it. Low-fat chocolate milk is a great way to deliver protein and carbs to a body in need (postworkout). An endurance athlete I was not, but I figured if drinking chocolate milk after intense runs would help those guys absorb protein better, it could also work for someone looking to build muscle in the gym. The article also helped me understand for the first time the process of how

Check out this "Anabolic Circle of Gains"

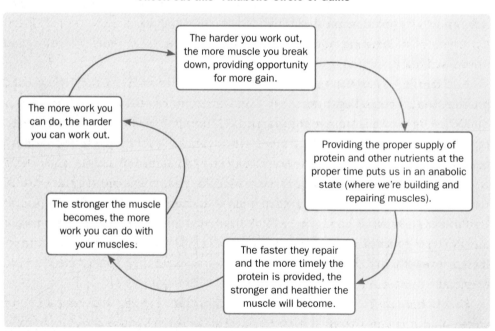

The harder you work out, the more muscle you break down, providing opportunity for more gain.

The more work you can do, the harder you can work out.

Providing the proper supply of protein and other nutrients at the proper time puts us in an anabolic state (where we're building and repairing muscles).

The stronger the muscle becomes, the more work you can do with your muscles.

The faster they repair and the more timely the protein is provided, the stronger and healthier the muscle will become.

our bodies breaks down and uses protein. Turns out that chocolate milk helps the absorption process because the extra carbs and sugar in the chocolate help protein reach the muscles faster, therefore providing better recovery results. So, better recovery equals better gains, all for the exact same amount of work.

Supplements: The Ultimate Shortcut

As my education continued, I began to truly understand the impact and benefit of supplements on building muscle. The fact is, a good workout without proper diet, nutrition, and supplementation is like driving a car without a steering wheel. You may know where you want the car to go, you just don't know how to get it there. Once you start learning how to use supplements correctly, you'll be full speed ahead without any extra work!

In a matter of months, my body transformed into a lean, mean block of solid muscle. Soon, others began to notice and wanted in on the secret. First was my buddy J.D., to whom I'll forever be grateful. Thinking they might give us an advantage over our peers, he was always game to try the various harebrained schemes I concocted. Crazy as some of these ideas were, they actually worked; and after a while, he, too, began to see enhanced results. For nearly a whole year after every workout, we'd run into our cells, grab a glass of chocolate milk and some peanut butter–and-jelly sandwiches for added whole-food nutrients, then meet in the wing to wine and dine on our "superfoods" and discuss the various forms of physical torture we'd just put ourselves through, and how we might make these efforts even more productive.

Slowly but surely, people noticed our gains, and they began asking what we were doing and why. Clearly it worked, but they were unconvinced that this recovery snack could be the secret ingredient. So I began the process of educating my peers on how supplements worked. Once I did, our wing was forever changed. Before I knew it, more and more people started walking around with a glass of milk after our scheduled gym or outdoor track times. By the end of summer, 15 to 20 people (a quarter of the wing) could be seen walking around after their workouts with their chocolate milk and PB & Js. I loved it!

The Dusk Before Dawn

Then, without warning, disaster struck! My face and back began to break out in permanent red hives. Was it my new sunscreen? A different fabric softener? My shampoo? I tried everything to get rid of this problem, an issue I'd had only once before, back when I was locked up in county jail away from the sun for nearly two years. Out went the sunscreen, I started to wash my clothes by hand, and I threw away my shampoo. I couldn't go to a doctor due to the fact that, for all intents and purposes, "medical care" does not exist in prison, hence my extensive troubleshooting. Nothing worked. Never did it occur to me that the six bags of powdered milk I was consuming per week might be the cause of this problem. It was my last option, the only thing I hadn't yet tried to replace.

Reluctantly, painfully, slowly . . . I let go of my milk fix. It was traumatic. I needed a support group, I needed . . . HELP! Over the course of the next few weeks, my gains diminished, a big blow to my efforts, but so, too, did my hives. Milk, it turned out, was the culprit. My new best friend had betrayed me. Beat down, depressed, and defeated . . . I gave in. Back to the meat I went. These products, while still good, simply didn't have the same effect, but milk had to go. My workouts suffered and my morale slumped. What was I to do?

Then, from nowhere, a ray of light! Word of protein bars (pure whey protein!) permeated the air. J.D. had been lobbying for them and word had it that negotiations were being conducted. Could it be possible? Could the morbidly obese people who ran the prison canteen, people who couldn't even speak their own name correctly and had no understanding of healthy food, be considering selling protein bars? Could J.D. pull it off? Wait, were these things even any good?

Back to the books I went. This was serious business! After studying everything I could get my hands on about protein, its various sources, and its various forms, I was sold. While protein bars wouldn't digest quite as quickly as a shake, they were still pretty amazing. In fact, I'm eating one as I write this sentence. They're just that good! With 20 grams of whey protein, 24 grams of complex carbs, and 5 grams of good fats, the Quest Bars they chose to sell us in prison were by far the best supplement I'd ever had. Come to think of it, until my release at the age of 29, they were the only *real* supplement I'd ever had. What's even more amazing is the fact that, from what I can see, these Quest protein bars are basically the best bars on the market today. Super lean and super healthy. Glad that canteen got one thing right!

After nine months of semisparse use (the canteen would only sell us 10 a week, so I could not get nearly as many bars as I would have liked), my body was as big as ever, but I had lost about seven pounds of fat, weight I didn't even know I had to lose! I was more ripped then I ever thought possible. I was eating these things like candy, and at first, people thought I was nuts to spend all my money on something with only 20 grams of protein. Once again, I had to reeducate everyone, and soon enough, at the end of rec time, it was milk and protein bars galore! We were all getting healthier and finally seeing real gains!

Now that I'm free there are so many options. Even so, I still use these protein bars throughout the day to help me meet my predetermined protein requirements while also staying in an anabolic state. I have also recently incorporated the use of protein powders. There are two main reasons for this. The first is a simple matter of practicality. Like most people, I cannot afford adequate amounts of protein in the bar form. Based on what I've seen, it generally costs about two times or more for a bar than what you could get in powder form. Crazy, right? I guess that's the price you pay for convenience. Imagine all the money you could save here if you're consuming over 100 grams of protein supps a day. The second, as noted earlier, involves how fast one's body absorbs the protein. If you're looking for a postworkout muscle rejuvenator, the solidity of the bar will *slow down* the absorption rate, and you may miss out on part of that all-important feeding window.

So you may be wondering, what's up with these protein powders? Are they good for us and can they be considered "natural," even though they've been processed down to powder form? Let's take a look at whey protein, often considered the gold standard in supplementation. Whey is derived from milk, which is 80 percent casein and 20 percent whey. In a nutshell, manufacturers extract the whey and concentrate it into its purest form. So essentially what you're getting is this: fast-acting, easily absorbable protein with no unnecessary carbs or fats, which would accumulate as unwanted calories while also slowing down the rate of protein absorption (incredibly important in postworkout recovery). Essentially, whey protein is a natural product taken to its limits by stripping it of the things our body doesn't want or need, thus leaving us what we desire most: lean muscle. Interestingly enough, whey is, in this sense, processed. However, it's not processed in the way people usually speak of these foods, which are generally full of odd chemicals and foreign substances meant to improve taste and shelf life. This is just one example of why it's not good to talk in absolutes and say never consume ANY processed foods.

Now back to that shake we spoke of earlier. Sorry, everyone, I wasn't referring to the ice cream–laden, full-fat version. Instead, I'm referring to a protein shake— the kind beloved by athletes and bodybuilders around the world!

This form of supplementation is incredibly healthy, often all natural, and is readily accessible in a choice of easy-to-mix flavors. You've got a healthy, filling, low-calorie meal. Even better is that you can then supplement this supplement by adding anything you like to meet an endless list of needs: greens, omegas, nuts, veggies, juices, frozen fruits, yogurt, you name it. In fact, one delicious shake could easily meet more of your essential daily dietary needs than your entire current diet. Think about that. Oh, and did I mention it could also cost less while also being easier to prepare? Yep, sounds like a win, win, win to me. I'll take two, please!

The reason these shakes are so good for you, beyond the fact that they offer very specific proteins, is that they can keep you in an anabolic state (where you're growing muscle) without exceeding the calorie requirements often associated with their whole-food forms. Of course that's before all the added ingredients, which only add nutritional value (if you choose carefully). These proteins also digest faster or slower in your body depending on which type of protein you've opted for, which will help you meet key protein-synthesis "windows," like postworkout or while you sleep.

Makers simply extract the proteins from various naturally occurring sources such as milk, egg, soy, or beef and condense them into one easily digestible powder. Once mixed with water, OJ, tea, or any other liquid for that matter, you're in business. It's that easy.

After much research on this subject, I've narrowed the world of supplements down to three main categories:

- Daily Supplements
- Preworkout Supplements
- Postworkout Supplements

Of course I didn't always know this. In prison your diet is heavily restricted, the food is bad, and there are basically NO readily available supplements. Looking back on the measures I used in an effort to "supplement" my diet while in prison, all I can do is shake my head! Although sound in theory, it is quite amazing the lengths I had to go to in order to develop a body that appeared worthy of all the work I'd been putting into it.

In contrast, my journey into this world of supplementation as a free man was swift, and I can see how it would be easy to become overwhelmed with all the enticing options. That said, I have found one brand that I truly enjoy, Optimum Nutrition. I am currently taking Gold Standard and Hydrowhey, which I often mix with Optimum's casein supplements. For the lean, athletic look without too much bulk, this seems to fit the nutritional profile just about right. If you're looking to bulk up, you may need something with a few more carbs and a bit more protein, but that is not the look or the feel I want to achieve with my body. So far as normal, everyday protein supplementation goes, this regimen or something comparable should work just fine for everyone . . . especially because I find these products to be priced competitively.

The following is my list of ideal fundamental supplements. Now, remember these are SUPPLEMENTS, meant to "supplement" your diet, not to replace healthy eating. They ADD to those areas where it's difficult to fulfill all your daily nutritional needs. Also, be sure to keep in mind that it's just as important WHEN you use these supplements as it is *how much* you use and the *type* you use. Studies suggest your body can only absorb about 20 to 50 grams of protein at a time, so be careful not to take in a whole lot more than that. Much more of any one kind will just convert into excess calories.

My Ideal Supplements
- Whey protein—Builds and feeds muscle
- Casein protein—Builds and feeds muscle
- BCAAs (branched-chain amino acids)—help build muscle while preventing breakdown
- Juice plus fruit-and-veggie pills—Good source of vitamins and minerals
- Low-dose multivitamin—Ensures your body replaces essential nutrients
- Probiotic—Good for improving digestive-tract health
- Ubiquinol or coenzyme Q10—"An ally against aging" as Dr. Oz says. Too many benefits to list.
- Omega-3s from flaxseed oil—Great for joints, skin, blood-fat levels, and much more
- Preworkout—Provides extra energy and endurance to help you work harder in the gym

My Ideal Usage Upon Waking (As Soon as You Get out of Bed)
- 25 grams whey protein
- 25 grams casein protein
- Flaxseed oil
- Ubiquinol
- Probiotic supplement in pill form

Breakfast (One to Two Hours After Waking)

- Low-dose multivitamin
- Juice plus fruit-and-veggie pills

Preworkout (30 Minutes Before Gym)

- 20 grams whey protein and/or a preworkout with whey protein
- 5 grams BCAAs

Postworkout (Immediately After Gym)

- 25 grams whey protein
- 25 grams casein protein
- 5 grams BCAAs

Night

- 25 grams whey protein
- 25 grams casein protein

Above is the ideal plan for me. Since it's nice and balanced, hopefully it will help you grow and achieve *your* goals. Keep in mind, this is just one example of an endless arrangement of supplementation plans, so try it, tweak it where necessary, and find out what works best for you. As you can see, I like to keep things simple and natural. It feels good to my body and eases my mind, since chemicals and highly processed junk scare the crap out of me. This is about health after all, and health to me equals longevity.

I'm sure my plans will evolve in the years to come as I continue to educate myself about the world of supplements. Just recently I've been learning about what preworkouts to take and what they do for your body. There are generally a lot of interesting ingredients in these things, far too many to list here, so my advice would be to get busy, do your research, and most important, be careful. Following my own advice, I have found Cellucor's C4, the M.A.S.S. Project's BUZZERK, and Optimum Nutrition's preworkouts to be quite good. These three supps give me the edge I need and can be used for a variety of training needs and goals. I enjoy the BUZZERK for cardio and circuit training, Cellucor for going hard in the gym and attempting to maximize gains, and ON's pres for my maintenance periods.

Whether you choose to use these preworkouts and whatever your ultimate physical goals, it's important to remember this basic plan. In tandem with your workout and diet, it will help you build muscle and burn fat in ways I found to be beyond amazing. So what are you waiting for . . . start supplementing!

The Take

- You break muscles down in the gym and build them back up in bed.
- When it comes to supplements, don't get overwhelmed; keep it simple.
- Research what you put into your body.
- Supplementation can and should be as close to natural as possible.
- Supplements are intended to fill the void that whole foods alone can't reach.
- Optimize your supplementation by using them when you wake up, before you work out, after you work out, and before bed.
- Protein is king!
- Remember, NOT all proteins are created equal. Choose your sources wisely!

- You can accelerate your gains by properly resting and recovering.

- Sleep is incredibly important, especially if you are following an active lifestyle and training hard. Aim for approximately eight hours nightly.

- Knowing when and how to apply these principles can save you time, effort, and energy. Muscles are primarily composed of water and protein. We need lots of both if we wish to develop lean muscle mass. Proper timing of your supplements will boost your gains.

7

The waist is a terrible thing to mind.

—ZIGGY (TOM WILSON)

Abs

We're here, everyone! The holy grail of the fitness world, the most sought-after destination, the embodiment of sexual appeal, the apex of our aesthetic goals . . . our abs! Oh, how I hate the abs. Not in the "oh crap, it's abs day again" kind of way, but in the *"rawrrr* . . . I just punched a hole in the wall" kind of way. Nothing, and I mean NOTHING, frustrates me nearly as much in my years-long quest to reach my peak physical form than that evasive six-pack. I. HATE. ABS . . . or at least I used to.

For years, the attempt to get well-defined abs was the bane of my existence. No matter what I tried, they still wouldn't show. Five-minute abs, dance abs, judo abs, whatever abs, you name it abs, it never worked. So for a long time I resigned myself to the deflating belief that abs just weren't going to happen for me. I had a decent core, just no definition. No . . . raw muscle.

I think for the most part, we all feel this way at some point in time. We all have weaknesses—you know, those parts of the body that just won't develop correctly no matter what we do. It may be your arms or your chest, but almost universally, it's the abs as well. The question then becomes, why is this? Are they really that stubborn? The answer . . . NO! The reality is that we just hate what we don't understand. Abs are complicated, and most fitness books explain the science behind them in increasingly complex terms. Because of this, many people come to despise the abs.

Not us, though, we're taking control! Yep, I'm going to help you get that washboard stomach. Hell, if I did it with these stingy things my genetics stuck me with, you can, too!

My breakthrough moment was hard-won. It came after years of research, when I made one discovery. If you want to attain sculpted abs you have to use . . . wait for it . . . WEIGHT!

Sound familiar? As you already know from our conversations earlier in this book, basic physics/physiology has shown us that in order to grow muscle, we must stimulate it with . . . you guessed it . . . weight. Like all other muscles, the unfortunate reality is that little resistance = little growth. The problem is that most people, myself included, tend to develop a severe case of amnesia regarding this basic fact when it comes to developing our abs. It's as though we've collectively fallen victim to the false assumption that abs are the only part of the body capable of growth without the aid of extra force. Check out most of the ab workouts and you'll see what I mean. It's staggering how many of them leave out that incredibly important ingredient, resistance.

Turns out that all those abs books, videos, and outlandish workouts have missed a lot. While adding weight *resistance* was the most pivotal discovery in my quest for developing the abs I'd always dreamt about, the ultimate reality was that . . . GETTING ABS TAKES A MULTIPRONGED APPROACH. Without understanding and adhering to several principles at once, your chance of attaining the abs of your dreams is about as likely as winning the lottery without buying a ticket. It's not going to happen. No wonder I, as well as everyone I knew, hated abs. Unlike the lottery, however, when you enter this game, your chances of success are infinitely greater. The more you play by the rules, the greater those odds go up.

This is where education once again becomes our best friend. Let's wipe the slate clean on everything we think we know about abs and begin a new chapter on our "core" fundamentals.

Core Development

I've named this chapter Abs, but this is really a chapter dedicated to your core. What's that? Essentially, it's the sum total of key muscle groups: lower back, transverse abdominals, rectus abdominals, obliques, and the all-important hip flexors, which collectively make up . . . you guessed it . . . our core. You want abs? Well, get to work on your core.

Our core's significance is similar to that of the car's frame or the stitching on a baseball. I like to think of it as the superhighway that connects our whole body. In essence, the core is what keeps all the parts of our bodies functioning in unison, while also taking on the important task of protecting our spines, organs, and other parts by acting as a kind of rigid internal girdle. A solid core also makes us stronger in everything from our squats to our bench presses, while also defining the waist, thus slimming us down and leaving us with an aesthetically pleasing V-shaped torso (much like a real-life girdle).

First, we must address the cold hard truth. In order to get abs you can actually see and be impressed with, you must first understand that it won't happen until you're at or below 12 percent body fat. Taking this into account, you can easily see that doing ab workouts alone will never get you the abs of your dreams. As the saying goes, "Abs are made in the kitchen, not in the gym." Nothing will hold you back more in your quest to develop abs than an ineffective diet.

So where do you start? In order to develop amazing abs, I believe you need to implement three important factors, listed in order of priority: (1) a steady diet; (2) a regular workout program; and (3) a structured cardio regimen. Without these three elements as part of your everyday lifestyle, you can do sit-ups until you're blue in the face and you'll never see a single ab. That's why I've placed this chapter so far back in this book, right there in the nosebleed section! If your goal is to see abs and you've not first developed the essentials mentioned in the previous chapters, YOU'RE WASTING YOUR TIME.

Now, at this point it's also important to note that once you're under 12 percent body fat, you'll likely see abs no matter how much you've exercised them. How many of us know one of those genetically fortunate people, somebody who clearly doesn't work out, yet one who happens to be sporting a decent set of abs on a rail-thin frame? Frustrating doesn't even begin to describe it. I've known quite a few of these individuals in my life, and, in full disclosure, I was kind of one of them for quite some time. This look always seemed a bit off to me, though. Until recently I could never quite figure out why. Then it hit me. There's a difference between "skinny abs" and what I refer to as "real abs." Take a look at two people of comparable size, one who works out and the other who doesn't, and you'll soon see what I mean. Which would you rather look like? They look completely different, right?

Once you've eliminated the layer of fat covering your abs through a well-balanced, nutritional diet, it's time to begin a regular training program, one that will incinerate existing fat reserves while building thicker, more profound abs. It's also important to find the cardio program that will continue to burn what's left around the edges of your core. Just as we needed to get our diets in order, we must also take the time to optimize our weight-training and cardio programs so we can align our efforts in the most effective way possible, thus demolishing fat and giving us the best overall results.

With all the energy and effort we've been putting into your improved body just to get to this point, it'd be a shame to stick to some tired, old workout formula from the past. That's why we're going to go big. If you want to see gains, you gotta put

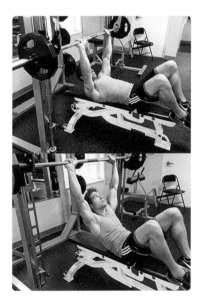

Smith Machine Crunch

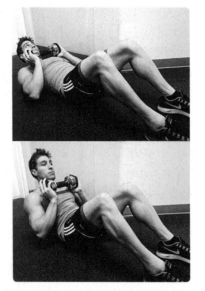

Weighted Crunch

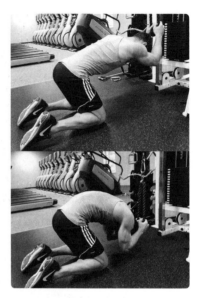

Cable Crunch

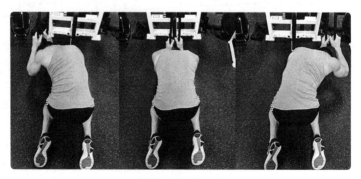

Cable Side Crunch

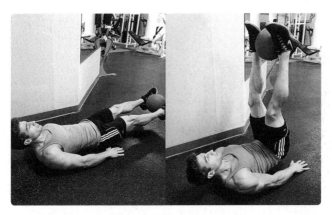

Weighted Leg Raise

in the work. No Richard Simmons nonsense here! We're going heavy, we're going hard, and we're going often! There are several workouts that can be shoehorned in at this point, many of which will hopefully build the big, thick, aesthetically pleasing abs I worked so hard to get, but these are the main ones I found most effective.

Trust me, these moves WILL separate you from the crowd. As you can see, a lot goes into creating a decent set of abs. While this may seem a bit daunting at first, I can assure you, it's far better than being misled by the latest fad promising a six-pack with minimal work and in minimal time. Mark my words, this crap almost inevitably guarantees your failure.

As far as I'm concerned, a six-pack is a great goal and there's no doubt in my mind that we can all obtain one. All we have to do is let go of our unrealistic expectations, start making small changes, put in a little work, and accept the steady pace of positive progress that comes with time and consistency. Those Hollywood bodies we all admire were not created overnight. So start making changes now, put in the necessary work, and get ready to show off come beach season . . .

The Moves

Once again, just as in Chapter 3, your ab regime will be split between main moves and interchangeable moves, only this time we'll also be throwing in a few "core specific" moves that will neither be heavy nor ab centric but instead will be more focused on building that overall superhighway core strength.

Weighted Main Moves	Interchangeables	Core Specifics
Smith Machine Weighted Crunch	Hanging Leg Raise	Swiss Ball Plank
Cable Crunch	Hanging Leg Side	Swiss Ball Jackknife
Side Cable Crunch	Reverse Crunch	Swiss Ball Pike
Medicine Ball Crunch	Lying Leg Raise	Side Plank
Weighted Leg Raise	V-Up	Plank
	Regular Crunch	Mountain Climber
	Raised Leg Crunch	Static Back Extension
		Prone Cobra
		Oblique Crunch

The Plan

Below is an example of my typical week of core training. As you may recall, the charts in Chapter 3 that detail the Big Six Moves fitness plan all had a specific spot for abs work. Because of its importance, weight is used on two of the three days. Sometimes I'll go heavy on the third day, but this can be a bit much for one week, and the last thing you want to do is take yourself out of the game by overtraining. That's why on the third day I try to do more core-specific workouts to better prevent injury and boost overall strength.

With this particular regimen, you're starting with the heavy lifts so you don't wear yourself out. This ensures that you hit the proper number of reps with correct form (remember poor form only sets you up for injury). On these, your rest time should be around 60 seconds in between sets.

The second exercise in each workout will be our interchangeable. These are more moderate movements where both form and function are essential to complete the full range of motion. Less rest time is required (approximately 30 to 45 seconds), since these movements are generally easier. If you need more rest time on a few, as I often do on hanging leg sides, then feel free to improvise.

Last, but certainly not least in this workout, are your core-specific moves. These are my favorite and you'll soon see why. They may not seem too difficult at first, but after a set or two you'll feel an incredible burn that immediately says you're on the right track! I always perform these exercises last because they seem to highlight what I've already done and give me a big sense of overall accomplishment. Rest for about 30 seconds between sets and on the last one either hold the plank for as long as possible or perform as many reps as possible. If you're anything like me, you'll love the sense of pushing yourself, and it'll make you love being finished with the workout even more! There are many other options, but I've listed what I consider the most important for you. Have fun and mix it up. But no matter what . . . YOU GOTTA GO HEAVY.

My Three-Day Core Workout

Remember, just pick one or two movements from each section for each day and do your thing. There aren't a whole lot of moves I feel just HAVE to be done each week, but the Smith machine crunch, cable crunch, leg raise, and plank do fall into that special category. As far as I've been able to tell, nothing works better at building muscle while simultaneously obliterating fat and sucking in your gut. So here it is.

Day 1

Exercise	Sets	Reps
Smith Machine Crunch	5	10
Hanging Leg Side	5	10
Regular Crunch	5	20
Swiss Ball Jackknife	5	10
HIITs x 5 +5-minute warm-up and cooldown		

Day 2

Exercise	Sets	Reps
Cable Crunch	3	20
Side Cable Crunch	3	20
Leg Raise	5	20
Oblique Crunch	5	10
Swiss Ball Pike	5	10
HIITs x 5 +5-minute warm-up and cooldown		

Day 3

Exercise	Sets	Reps
Weighted Leg Raise	5	10
Reverse Crunch	5	10
V-Up	5	10
Swiss Ball Plank	5	1 min.
Side Plank	5	30 sec.
Static Back Extension	5	30 sec.
30 minutes steady-state cardio		

One more quick tip! As you can see above, I often throw in a quick interval session (the HIITs we spoke of in Chapter 4) on core day. It's time efficient, and I feel like it really works my abs just a little harder than normal. I haven't read any science on this, but it works for me and that's all that really matters. This is important to note, since much of finding a personally appropriate workout functions this way. Studies and science are incomplete and they sure as heck aren't universal. If you discover something and it works for you, use it. I found this little trick in ninth grade when my physical education coach made me run a mile for each class I missed . . . due to playing in high school tennis matches. Figure that one out. On days we didn't have matches, I'd go to my last class of the day, PE; do sit-ups (what the coaches had us do couldn't even be considered exercise); and then hit the track while everyone else was leaving school. Although I was generally doing steady-state cardio exclusively, I still saw improvements and later found it would work with HIITs as well. Only difference is that I find HIITs to be more enjoyable as well as time effective. Amazing. Thanks, confused PE coach!

I also don't train abs two days in a row for two reasons: (1) You need proper time for rest and recovery; and (2) because the meat of our workouts, the Big Six, which you're hopefully using every other day, also works your core and therefore indirectly builds your abs. (Interestingly enough, this is where most bodybuilders get the mass that makes up their abs.) So I personally recommend alternating abs training with your regular workouts. It's what I find works best for me. Good luck!

The Take

- You don't have to hate abs because they *seem* complicated, you just have to understand them.
- Attaining abs requires a multipronged approach.
- In order to develop fully visible abs, you must first get your diet, workout, and cardio program in order.
- You must work your whole core—not just your abs.
- If you want abs with size and depth, you must train with weights.
- The main moves in Chapter 3 indirectly help build a solid core and noticeable abs.
- "Real" abs are made in the kitchen . . . AND the gym.
- In order for your abs to be truly visible, you need a body-fat ratio of 12 percent—or lower!

8

People don't stop moving when they get old.
They get old when they stop moving.

—WALTER M. BORTZ

Keep Moving

I'm someone who's always on the move. Always have been and likely always will be.

It all started long before prison when, as a kid, I loved recess and couldn't wait to go out and play. As soon as those doors opened to the outside world, I was gone. Football, basketball, soccer, kickball, tag, you name it, I was game. Sitting on the sideline with the "cool" kids seemed so odd and out of place to me. How could it possibly be cool to just sit there like a bump on a log in your Airwalks and Mossimo (the height of cool back then), and do nothing but talk to girls? *Eww* . . . it made no sense to me. Looking back, I guess the girls in elementary school didn't want stinky guys covered in sweat anyway. Who knew? It didn't matter, though; girls or no girls, I had to move.

Unfortunately, being in prison kind of took me back to my school days, and not in a good way. At school I often couldn't wait for the doors to open in between classes. In prison, I often found myself waiting for the doors to open, but to a far less inviting world. What I've found is that when you're out on the yard (think recess for prisoners), it's essential that you keep moving. If you're lazy in prison and listlessly milling around, as most people are, it's almost certain that the dope dealers, hustlers, and, worst of all, the predators will eventually make your acquaintance.

Not good. Those people are pushy, highly skilled, and dangerous. It's really just a matter of time before you become another lost, helpless victim. So how do you avoid dangerous people and even more dangerous situations when you're locked up?

Sure, you can try to hide out in your room, but unfortunately that never works. That's why I decided to stay in perpetual motion. It was a decision that came naturally to me, even though I really had no other options. I felt like a child playing peekaboo, one who believes that if you cover your eyes, they can't see you. The only difference was I kept hoping that if they couldn't keep up with me, then they'd eventually give up on me, thus making me effectively invisible. Fortunately, for me, it worked . . . most of the time.

Since I didn't hide and rarely hung out in groups (a whole other issue in itself), I was viewed very much as an individual and as my own man. Being who I wanted to be proved to be both a blessing and a curse. After a while, though, if you make it that long, you become sort of a fixture, one as overlooked as the miles of chainlink fence that surrounded the prison. Of course, this doesn't mean you're safe. You're NEVER safe, especially if you let your guard down. My fellow prisoners constantly played games and had nothing but time on their hands to come up with new ways of hustling people. Some would wait years for you to let your guard down, essentially playing a real-life game of chess. One false move and they'd have you in checkmate. Game over.

As the years passed, I just kept on moving and never stopped. I might have slowed down a little, but when I did, I kept my headphones on to further block out the guys around me. People knew I didn't like to be bothered, and if anyone wanted to chat I'd more often than not just pick up the pace. No games for me. I stuck to what I knew and kept it moving. It was a survival tactic, but it also helped me in my physical lifestyle. Whether you're in prison or outside in the free world, a sedentary lifestyle is just plain bad for you. So keep moving!

I'm sure you already know some of the benefits of continuous movement, but there's also a lot you likely haven't thought of. It alleviates depression, obesity, cardiovascular issues . . . the list goes on. From my own personal experience, I can tell you that my nonstop walking and activity also kept me slim, helped me feel great, and enabled me to avoid the dreaded 3 p.m. afternoon slump. So put down that coffee cup and energy drink . . . you don't need them. What you need to do instead is MOVE!

In fact, most of this book was written standing up! I wrote much of my first draft while still in prison and 90 percent of it was written while standing by my bunk (yes, we sleep on bunk beds in prison), and that's why it was tall enough. Sure, that's not a whole lot of movement, but it got me off my butt and made it easier for me to pace a few steps every now and then. Plus my posture was a whole lot better than if I were slumped over a desk. I won't even go into how screwed up my back is after almost 10 years on a prison bed.

It's difficult to convey just how incredibly important the act of continuous movement is in our lives, so to better illustrate my point, here's a great sentence I came across from Dr. Walter M. Bortz, who wrote *Living Longer for Dummies*, among other books on health and aging. He said, "If a pill existed that provided all of the health benefits that exercise provides, the whole country would be on it." Think about that. Those words certainly struck a chord in me. I truly believe that the vast majority of crap prescribed to us these days would be utterly unnecessary if people ate correctly, exercised, and took a long, hard look at themselves.

Now, I know some of you might be reading this and thinking, "I can barely make it round my block." Some of you know you're out of shape and the idea of intense exercise is daunting. But let me reveal an amazing fact. Which do you think burns more calories: running a mile or walking it? Well, guess what, the number of calories burned would be just about equal. Strange, right? I know, I thought the same way!

Sure, running may provide more cardiovascular and muscular benefits than walking, but the total amount of work done during a mile remains the same for both paces. So what we're really talking about here is a time issue. It generally takes around 16 minutes to walk a mile (thus burning about 100 calories) while it only takes eight minutes, half the time, to burn off those same 100 calories when running. So if you run for an hour, you are going to cover more ground and burn more calories than an hour of walking. But in a straight-up distance comparison, both modes are almost equally effective. My point? No matter what shape you're in, *get moving*. All exercise is beneficial. Don't stop yourself from getting started in the first place. Just do what you can and build on the momentum.

So once again, what are you waiting for? We all have ample opportunities in our lives to keep moving. Park a little farther away from work if you have to, work on your free throws, take a walk after dinner, or even pace back and forth instead of sitting the next time you're in your cell . . . oops, I meant on your cell. IT ALL ADDS UP! If I could stay active locked in a concrete block for over 20 hours a day, *you can too*!

Which Exercise Burns the Most Calories?

Okay, are you all ready for some interesting facts and figures? Listed below are some general activities and the number of calories they burn per hour. These are NOT exact figures, so don't go getting all pedantic on me! They're not even the same for each person. They're simply here to act as a guide and hopefully make you look at your active lifestyle a bit differently.

Calories Burned During One Hour Of:

Sleeping = 70	Jogging 5 miles per hour = 550
Sitting = 80	Basketball = 650
Bowling = 250	Tennis = 650
Walking 3 miles per hour = 330	Soccer = 650
Golf = 350	Ultimate Frisbee = 650
Biking 10 miles per hour = 350	Moderate stair stepper = 700
Hiking = 450	Running 7 miles per hour = 850
Moderate weight training = 450	Jumping rope = 900

The Take

- "A body in motion stays in motion." It's a fact that rings true in my life.
- Sustained, deliberate movement can help prevent obesity, depression, many cardiovascular issues, and a host of other conditions.
- Movement keeps you from sitting, which protects your back, hips, organs, and posture.
- Walking a mile burns almost as many calories as running a mile. All exercise is beneficial.

SO GET UP AND GET MOVING!

9

Success is a process, a quality of mind and a way of being.

—ALEX NOBLE

Be Consistent

By now you've hopefully noticed a common theme throughout the chapters in this book. Whether it's diet, exercise, cardio, recovery, or any of the other topics within these pages, the unifying theme that ties them all together is *consistency*.

Whether you want a fitness magazine–worthy body or just want to be healthier, your odds of success depend on your level of consistency. Consistency, consistency, consistency! Live it, learn it, love it! Write it down. Post it as a screensaver on your computer. Do whatever you can to never forget this essential element in your new life. You MUST hold yourself accountable.

As I was fighting to achieve a body that would help keep me safe and alive during my nearly 10 years in prison, it was my last two years of incarceration that would prove most productive. Sure, at this point I had developed a rock-solid foundation and, through education, slowly became aware of what my time and energies were best spent on. But what ultimately took me from being merely in good shape to looking like a *Men's Health* cover guy was first, believing in myself; second, believing in the program I'd developed; and third and most important of all, committing to consistency.

When it comes to health and fitness, I think this is where we as a society struggle most. We're all so desperate for instant gratification. With everything available in a matter of minutes in big-box stores or on the Internet, it's easy to forget that some of the best things in life take time.

In the case of our physical health, it takes a lot of time, both mentally and physically. It was only when I stopped looking for shortcuts to my physical goals that the answers became clear and results began to pile up. Once again, my willingness and desire to educate myself led me to my most important personal discovery about how our bodies grow and adapt.

Although I greatly respect the individuals who make a living flexing on stage and whose bodies are almost cartoonishly large, that look is not something I desire for myself. Instead of shunning this subculture's books, magazines, and workouts as many would likely do, though, I thought that there had to be a great deal of knowledge trapped within these publications that could be applicable to us mere humans. The same could be said about any professional sport/athlete, if one stopped and thought about it. For instance, I know I'll never be an NBA player, but that doesn't mean I can't adapt their jump shot technique or vertical leaping ability training.

Long story short, leaving my preconceived notions at the door has given me a wide range of ideas, methods, and philosophies that have improved my quality of life as well as made my training significantly more efficient. One thing that really struck me when reading about the big-dog bodybuilders—the Mr. Olympias and Mr. Universes—was that almost all were in their late twenties or early thirties when they were winning shows. "How could this be?" I thought. Shouldn't the younger guys be winning this stuff, as is the case with tennis, gymnastics, baseball, football, and basketball? I was confused. My only answer . . . more research.

After many hours of looking into this phenomenon, the answer came to me in an article about young up-and-comers in the sport. One particular article caught my eye, since it showcased an individual who had been working out for years with the explicit goal of gaining as much mass as possible. This man was larger than me and my last three cellies combined, yet he still had zero chance of winning against his older counterparts. Much to my surprise, this did not discourage him. He felt great about where he was physically and discussed how he would train certain areas of his body OVER THE NEXT FEW YEARS to gain the extra mass necessary to get where he needed to be. Needless to say, this amazed me. YEARS? What an incredible show of patience, understanding, and dedication.

We can take from this the inescapable fact that muscle generally takes a long time to grow and fat can take a long time to burn. That's just the way it is and that's if you're doing everything right. As the old expression goes: "Slow and steady wins the race." Once again, I had to accept what I could not change and change what I could. For me this meant not giving up when I didn't immediately see the unrealistic results I wanted and being content with the fact that I'd been making consistent gains. I came to accept that if I stuck to my plan, though it might take a while, I would get to where I needed to be.

Two years of consistency later, and here I am feeling better about myself than

I ever have before. Without even trying to lose weight, I dropped from 175 to 167 pounds, but I have remained larger than ever in terms of muscle (clearly losing fat I didn't even know I had) and was left more cut up than ever.

This may not seem like too big a deal, but by sticking to a diet and workout that didn't intrude too heavily on my life, I lost more than eight pounds of pure fat and, for the first time ever, had abs so defined that they look computer generated. What's amazing is that the only major thing I changed during the last two years was consistency. Instead of going for a few months, then stopping for a few months to play ball or be lazy, I showed up nearly every day, five to six days a week, for about an hour or so, and success simply happened. I didn't even push myself too hard. I just stuck to it, always eating healthy and never missing more than two weeks of exercise. I'm a new man and it's all because of one small change. I SHOWED UP.

The best part is, I keep thinking that I've reached my maximum potential, since I am incredibly satisfied with what I see in the mirror. Then two more months go by and I catch a glimpse of myself, and I am once again amazed at the progress I've made. I no longer worry about how to get in shape or how to keep the pounds off. I can now power through my workouts without overworking or becoming too regimented. All that's necessary now is keeping it simple, staying on track, sticking to the fundamentals I've outlined in this book, and being CONSISTENT! At this point, it's almost like I'm on autopilot. I've found great peace, eat quite a few cheat meals, and know my limits. I don't even worry about progress anymore. It just keeps coming!

The Take

- Consistency is the thread that unites all of your goals into one attainable package.
- Unrealistic expectations lead to letdowns and feelings of failure. You must be pragmatic.
- Many of the best things in life take time to develop.
- Muscle takes time to grow and fat takes time to burn.
- Stop looking for shortcuts and success will find you.
- Remember, slow and steady wins the race.

JUST SHOW UP!

10

You are not your circumstances. You are your possibilities.

—OPRAH WINFREY

Belief and Willpower

If there's one fundamental characteristic that successful people share, it's a healthy dose of self-esteem. Regardless of what life throws their way, they have an ingrained belief that they will be able to gain control of their environment and do whatever they want in life. While this key component is necessary for just about any situation we may encounter on this earth, it is all the more important in a maximum-security prison where strength of character can literally mean the difference between life and death.

Until I found myself thrust into this decade-long nightmare, I had no idea that I had such self-belief. To this day, I still don't know where it came from: a loving family, a positive childhood, perhaps a naive hope in the inherent good of the world? Who knows? All I do know is that regardless of where my self-esteem came from, I'm glad I had it. I believe without a doubt that it was one of the key factors that kept me out of harm's way. The most likely reality is that I lucked into the whole "fake it till you make it" philosophy, since I knew I didn't stand a chance against many of these hardened convicts. It worked, though . . . at least well enough until I was able to get a handle on things.

That's essentially what this whole book is about. NEVER GIVE UP, KEEP PUSHING!

I'm a fan of Dr. Wayne Dyer and especially his book *Your Erroneous Zones*. In the book, Dyer explains that we control our thoughts, and therefore it is we who control our emotions. Thoughts lead to feelings, feelings lead to actions. It's much like a self-fulfilling prophecy where you will become what you think you are. In essence, we are in complete control of our destiny, the sole manipulator of our universe. It's all a matter of what thoughts and feelings you allow to control your reality.

Let's take that idea a bit further. I've noticed that I often feel at my best when I accomplish specific objectives. We are largely a goal-driven society, with clearly defined paths to success. Do your homework, study hard, and make good grades. Practice your jump shot, work hard at the gym, and win ball games. Accomplishment and growth are the secrets to happiness. It's an important realization that can be invaluable when it comes to our own health and fitness.

This brings me to one of the biggest roadblocks people encounter when trying to improve their fitness. How many people (myself included at times) have tried getting into shape, only to become disillusioned and throw in the towel? If this is something you find yourself nodding your head yes to, it's okay, you're far from alone.

The problem, once again, becomes that insatiable need for instant gratification. I strongly believe that all good things take time, and though we may not see all the hard work and sacrifice that goes into other people's incredible accom-plishments, trust me, they put the work in! Take professional athletes for example. In his book *Outliers*, Malcolm Gladwell explores a time commitment that lends perspective to getting into shape. Becoming competitive at the highest levels of athletics (or at any endeavor) requires dedicating approximately 10,000 hours of time to pure practice. No games, scrimmages, or workouts, just PRACTICE. How crazy is that? Sure, I'd love to be a pro tennis player, but do I really want to spend three hours a day for the next ten years on nothing but practice in my desire to fulfill this dream? Ahh . . . no thanks. You, too, likely don't aspire to be a world champion, but the principle still applies. We have to be willing to put in the work. There are no shortcuts.

What's important to note is that we can break free of this trap, this desire to succeed without struggle. Whether you've realized it or not, the simple act of shed-ding light on unrealistic expectations as we have just done has already kick-started the growing process. An internal battle within you has likely begun, and whatever the outcome, you can only gain from this newfound knowledge. Having initiated the growing process by taking our detrimental, unrealistic thoughts out of the basement and thrusting them into the light, we can begin to nurture what we've taken from this newfound knowledge and use it as the impetus to inspire and create lasting growth! By shedding those UNREALISTIC EXPECTATIONS that have been holding us down, we can now take our time and make realistic, achievable, short-term, as well as a few long-term, goals.

Now, we must take a moment to figure out what exactly constitutes a realistic expectation. Always more questions! Keep questioning! It's part of the grow-ing process: QUESTIONS = understanding; understanding = growth; growth = progress; and progress = MEETING OUR GOALS. Therefore, asking QUESTIONS ultimately results in MEETING OUR GOALS. And to answer the question of what constitutes a realistic expectation: Just as you cannot count your reps before your sets are done, you cannot count on attaining or achieving anything until the hard work has been done. Believe in yourself and do the work that you know you're capable of, and you can open up a whole new world of possibilities.

With that out of the way, we can focus on what is, to me, the crux of this chapter and probably of this book. Come to think of it, in many ways it might just be the crux of my life: WILLPOWER. Before we make our goals, we have to understand that without the necessary allotment of willpower to dedicate ourselves to some form of consistency, attaining our goals will be incredibly difficult (if not impossible). When it comes to our overall health, willpower means you continually choose to make the best decision, regardless of what's going on around you. In my life, this has meant that no matter what the daily vicissitudes, which were plentiful in a maximum-security prison, there are things that must always be done: Eat the appropriate food, never diverging too far from your optimal diet. Stay with the books, continually looking for new and exciting ways to liven up your routines. Always go to the gym or get some form of exercise, whether it be walking, running, or simply pushing weights around until one day your peace of mind comes back around . . . which it will. The goal is simply to stay on task, always moving forward, always improving, and never getting too far behind.

At first I thought willpower and self-belief were the same thing, but they're not. Many people believe in themselves, but they often fail to achieve the level of success they thought possible. Why? They don't take action! Willpower is action, the propellant necessary to get the job done. This action, this . . . overwhelming force is ultimately what separates the mere good from the GREAT! It is the key ingredient you'll find in risk takers, business leaders, top athletes, movie stars, and the successful all around the world. Belief (thought) driven by willpower (action) makes you unstoppable.

So how do we get to the point of shifting willpower into action? Through the thoughts we choose to believe, of course. While willpower does rely on a great foundation of belief and self-confidence, the difference between willpower and self-confidence comes at that point where we choose to separate ourselves from the masses of what I call pseudo-self-confident believers, those who don't apply action to their overconfident thoughts. Belief without the willpower to act on your thoughts is nothing but a lie people tell themselves to comfort and conceal their underlying self-doubt. What's obvious when you take a look around is that nearly everyone you see hasn't yet reached his or her full potential. I certainly haven't. You may attribute this to laziness, as I once did, but I now think it comes from fear: fear of wasting time, fear of looking stupid, or worse, fear of failure. As Dr. Wayne Dyer once said, "You can avoid ever having to fail by avoiding all activities that involve some risk. In this way you never have to come face-to-face with your self-doubt." This quote couldn't be more true. How many times have you met people who want something so intensely that you'd think they'd do anything to acquire that object, skill, or relationship—but because they were afraid of not succeeding, they never even attempted to fulfill that desire? Now, how many times has that person been you?

I can't count how many times I've heard people say they wish they were in shape, then did nothing to help themselves get there. When I asked why they didn't hit the weights or join that yoga class, it almost always came down to fear, and even though they were plainly saying it to me, they couldn't see it themselves. "I don't know how," "I'll look like a fool," "Everyone else is so far ahead of me" . . . the list goes on and on. Excuses! Fears! Nothing more, nothing less. LET IT GO!

It took me many years to understand this. Life in prison for me was a series of "highs," if you could call them that, and "lows" affecting my mental state on a daily basis. I was oftentimes lost and allowed my level of anxiety, as well as my diet, to get out of control. Things would be going along smoothly when out of nowhere the courts would make some illogical decision, plunging me into negativity. The first thing to go was my diet. My fears of uncertainty ultimately took control and drove me into a state of survival, thus "relieving" me of any duty I had toward my regular eating habits. Soon after, my energy would suffer due to a lack of nutrition, which would subsequently cause a deterioration in my workouts. Instead of doing the simple things to maintain all of the hard work I'd been putting into my health, I, like so many of us, slowly let things slide. I became captive to my fears and self-doubt. Without even realizing it, this degenerative lifestyle soon became a cycle that eventually fed off of itself, pushing me further and further away from my goals. For many, these temporary setbacks soon become a permanent lifestyle, and that's how people lose years from their lives.

It doesn't have to be that way, though. If you're one of the lucky ones, you may have avoided this pitfall. I have, however, seen it all too often, and I can only testify to what I know and have experienced in life. At first I thought I had no fears, hell, I was handling my own in prison. This wasn't the case, though. Fears come in all shapes and sizes. I'd love to explain them here, but whole books have been written on this very subject. All I know is that if you feel like you have no fears, really examining what you think and feel could change your entire life. With an understanding of our basic thought processes, both good and bad, and a healthy dose of willpower, we can blunt the effects of negativity, take control of our lives, and turn that cycle around.

Of my relatively short three decades here on earth, moments of inaction are the only ones I truly regret. I'm talking about times when I remained inactive due to fear or because I was "too busy," or "not in the mood." It was all crap. What it really boiled down to was insecurity. Once I changed how I felt about the possibility of not succeeding on my first try, my life changed. I've since learned to juggle, play guitar, perform handstand push-ups, get into better physical shape than pretty much anyone I know, and of course write this book. These are all things I wouldn't have even attempted if I hadn't first allowed belief to triumph over self-doubt and allowed my inner willpower to beat out my fears and laziness.

Even as I write these very words, I still feel a bit apprehensive about how this book will be received, but the reality is it no longer matters. I've given it all that I've got, and I hope and believe these words will help someone, somewhere, to think about life and health and fitness in a different way. Ultimately, the very act of writing this book is an accomplishment I never thought possible five years ago. Writing these final words has already brought me the fulfillment of meeting a major goal, one that, no matter what, I will keep with me for the rest of my life.

Let me leave you with these final words. The last 10 years of my life have been in many ways a nightmare. It is hard to describe just how difficult the years were. But I can confidently take with me the knowledge that I left prison stronger, faster, and smarter than I could ever have dreamed. I made that happen! Me! I willed it into existence! The neat thing about this is nothing in this world can stop you from making big changes in your life, too.

I believe that anything is possible if we only have the courage to begin. So start with this book. Implement little changes to your diet, your workout, and your studies. Once you taste success, try those same skills in another area of your life . . . then keep on going until you've conquered the world!

Believe in yourself and take action!

The Take

- Belief (thought), followed up with willpower (action), mixed with a little determination can accomplish anything.
- Begin building your belief and willpower by making small but significant changes. Adopt a "never say never" attitude.
- We CAN take control of our lives.
- Make small, easily achievable goals so that you can chart your progress.
- You have to be willing to put in the hard work.
- You and only you can make your dreams come true.
- Fake it till you make it if you have to.
- Don't fear failure; it's nothing but an inevitable step on the road to success. Only fear inaction.
- Stick to what you know works in hard times and you'll come out on the other side happier, healthier, and ready to take on the world!

The future belongs to those who believe
in the beauty of their dreams.

—ELEANOR ROOSEVELT

Conclusion

There you have it. Part of my story. Just a glimpse into what I've endured these past 10 years. A large portion of a series of books that will highlight the ins and outs of our criminal justice system, what it felt like to endure its inherent struggles, the story of me and my family coming into our own, the fight, the ultimate elation of success, and the peace that comes with attaining justice against all odds.

I sincerely hope this has been enough to whet your appetite until these other facets of my journey and my family's come together. I cannot express how much it means to me to be able to share this with you. Writing this book during the last five months of my incarceration was very cathartic. As the stress mounted in what could very well have been my last opportunity at redemption, I desperately needed an outlet. Not knowing if I'd ever be free again, or have another opportunity to prove my innocence, it came to be supremely helpful to write something that other people might be able to use in their daily lives. Not only the workouts, of course, but the story of love, family, and perseverance as well.

It's incredibly important for me to note that this is not all that I am. These things do not define me. My passion for health and fitness have helped me tremendously in all parts of my existence, and prison has clearly dominated much of my adulthood. This, however, is not all there is to life. Not for me at least. These two aspects of life are just part of what makes me . . . well, me.

While in prison I also came up with other tips, strategies, and techniques for growth and education in all areas of life. This "will to grow" evolved to become the primary philosophy I personally developed and adhered to for much of my time in prison. It's a philosophy rooted in not only pragmatism but also in the positive side of hate. This, of course, sounds contradictory, but if we are able to get over ourselves and push through the fickle pain of whatever ails us, we can then take the naturally occurring negative energy hate provides and channel it into positive action. If used in our daily lives, doors will inevitably open and the future will be ours. I believe we must alter the way we perceive hate, thus forcing us to look at negative energy as nothing but a fuel. It's there in all of us. It exists whether we want it to or not. Suppression and denial will do nothing but hurt us. We can either douse ourselves with this fuel and give in, thus burning away our dreams as most people do, or . . . we can be different. We can separate ourselves from the herd by creating an inner vehicle that uses this fuel to propel us to new heights. The choice is ours.

As you can gather, I'll be hard at work for the foreseeable future. What you've just read is simply part of what I've endured these past 10 years and how I endured it. There is much more to the story, and I look forward to sharing that with you in future books. While the scars from the recent past are fresher and deeper than I'm able to contemplate, I still feel as though I have much to offer this world. Beyond that, this is the best way I know to fight back, to express my individuality, and to show that I am a human being who might actually have a positive impact on people's lives, as so many of you have had on me. I am not a number! What could possibly be better than that, than taking control of your life, as well as giving back?

So this is me, Ryan William Ferguson, a person who has feelings, has dreams, and will do everything in his power to leave this world a better place than when he came into it. Nothing and no one will ever take that from me. EVER! I guess that's also, in some distorted way, the message I hope this book might convey. You'll get out of life only what you put into it, so why not be the absolute best you can be? Why let circumstances or other people or things we cannot control dictate our thoughts, our feelings, and, ultimately, our lives?

We can rise above this. Each and every one of us has the ability to take control of his or her own life no matter what the circumstances. I did it and this is just one of the ways, one of the single paths out of millions, that a person might take to enrich his or her time here on earth. As far as I can tell, we are ALL equal and the only thing that's separating those we admire from those we inspire is work. How much, how often, and how hard? It's just that simple.

Take a moment and ask yourself: How many times have I been inspired, yet never taken action? Until I considered this question personally, my life's purpose was largely unknown. It is only when I became inspired and then CHOSE to take action that doors began to open and the world's treasures were revealed to me— yes, even as a "nonperson" number in a world of grim oppression. To this day, that question is part of what motivates me to continue growing both mentally and physically. Inspiration is all around us—in the people we meet, the stories we hear, the lives we desire, or even a sunset that is so vibrant and elegant that it changes our perception of reality.

If we can harness this energy, and start by making small changes now, our goals will one day meet us along this path. This is precisely what I've done throughout the years when life was simply too difficult to shape by trying huge changes. One foot in front of the other was my path. Slowly, steadily, surely, my life improved. I felt better, I looked better, I had more confidence. This path became a lifestyle, and all the elements I needed for growth thankfully fell into place. Now that I've found my footing, it's become even more obvious to me just how useful are the subjects in this book. What's more, I know that together they create a force that cannot be stopped!

Once adopted and adhered to, these principles became second nature and it is then and only then that I realized how much easier it was getting and staying in shape than getting halfway into shape, falling back out, and then trying to get back in again. The willpower to keep persisting, to give whatever you've got through hard times, can make all the difference in the world. It's also what can make this way of life uncomplicated and satisfying.

Essentially, I'm saying that time spent in the gym or the kitchen is an incredibly important investment in your future, but . . . *it must be consistent.* One of the barriers to consistency in our current culture is what I call "the malaise of the two-season workout plan." For some reason, many people seem to behave very differently when it comes to their diet and exercise habits, depending on whether it's summer or winter.

This theory presupposes only two seasons, because people are generally concerned with looking good for the summer (the warm months) and not caring during the rest of the year (the cold months). Sound familiar? Can you count the people you know who work out religiously from about March to August, and then disappear for fall and the cold months? No wonder it's so difficult to get into shape when we only spend half a year trying. We have to get away from this destructive mentality.

That's why I don't believe in fad diets, or random multiweek workouts that promise "ripped abs" and "bulging biceps." Remember, there is no such thing as a short-term solution to a lifetime of consumption. What we have in the preceding chapters is a healthy, sustainable lifestyle that gives you better arms and abs than most people without having to torture yourself every six months just so you can fit into your swimsuit or take off your shirt. What's more, the multitude of benefits that accrue through this way of life, when compared to the purely aesthetic-driven culture of the two-season approach, are mind-boggling. Energy, endurance, disease prevention, self-esteem, quality of life, you name it. There's a good chance it's connected in some way to living a healthy, well-balanced, consistent lifestyle. And that, my friends, is why EVERYONE can benefit from this program. THIS IS A LIFESTYLE DIET!

So, as you can see, it's not about being perfect and it certainly isn't about "dieting." It's about understanding yourself, the science, and how things work for or against us. It's about understanding the important decisions that are yours alone, and the many conscious choices that will ultimately shape who you are and who you will become. Remember, this whole process is more of a marathon than a sprint, so pace yourself, take a few breathers to revel in the beauty of your journey, and, most important, enjoy the ride. This is your life after all.

To me, this is what life is all about: basking in the brilliance of what surrounds us and either taking advantage of, or better yet, creating your own opportunities. By combining the fundamentals of our most essential tools (diet, exercise, and education), and thus creating the foundation on which to build the future, your opportunities, like mine, will be plentiful. We just have to work hard and wait our turn.

Now that you know what this journey is all about, it's time to take control of your body, your mind, and . . . your life. Through AWARENESS and ACTION all things are possible. What you currently hold in your hands is awareness. It's now up to you to act!

Appendix

In this section I briefly explain the exercises presented in this book. This is just an overview of the fundamentals to get you started. I encourage further personal research into each of these exercises as you begin integrating them into your routines. For me, it is always best to see the moves completed in motion. Words on paper just don't quite translate to all of the minute details that go into each and every move. That's why I have created a free YouTube page and website, both, Ryan Ferguson Fitness, for you to be able to see the proper motion of each movement. I strongly recommend taking advantage of this valuable resource. Until then, you can follow these capsule descriptions as summaries.

Back Extension (Lower Back)
This move is great for strengthening your core and has been linked with the prevention of lower back injury, since it strengthens the muscles around your spine. However, if you experience back pain while attempting this move do not continue. To start, lie on your stomach on the floor with hands resting in front of you, palms down, feet out behind you. To engage, lift your arms and legs a few inches off of the floor at the same time and hold briefly at the top of the move. This is one rep. What's best—this move can be done anywhere!

Barbell Curl (Arms, Biceps)
Great move for getting better arms! Can be done with a wide grip for outer biceps and a narrower one for your inner bis. Either way is good and you will hit the majority of your muscles, so stick to what feels best! To perform, simply grab a barbell with a weight you

deem appropriate, something you can do at least 10 reps with; bend the knees a little while also keeping your back slightly arched; and curl the weight from about waist height up toward your chest. Be sure to keep elbows in and lower slowly for one rep. That's it!

Bench Press (Chest)

As described in Chapter 3, this is a great multijoint move that develops lean muscle. It's done lying on a bench with your feet on the floor and your shoulder blades pulled in toward the center of your back. Start with the weight above the center of your chest and slowly bring it down to the lower portion of your chest. Pause for a moment and push the weight back up to the top of the movement.

Bent-Over Row (Back and Arms)

This is one of my all-time favorite moves! Outside of a squat, I feel more muscles being worked when I do these than anything else. If you want a nice back, this is your move. With a barbell, lean over, bending knees slightly; then pull the barbell toward your upper waist and return arms to a downward position.

Box Jump (Legs)

The box jump is a great plyometric move, one that builds explosive leg strength while also providing cardiovascular benefits. Simply square up to a box of reasonable height (one to two feet for beginners). In one smooth motion, bend your knees into a quarter squat and jump on top of the box, much like a cat might, with both feet squarely on top. Step down quickly and repeat for five to 10 reps depending on intensity.

Bridge (Core, Glutes, and Obliques)

These are good calisthenics movements to build core strength. It's great to throw this exercise in at the end of a cardio or core day to build those inner nonsuperficial muscles. Lie flat on the floor with your knees bent shoulder width apart and your palms down on the floor beside you. Pushing up on your heels, lift your lower body off the ground while keeping your back straight. Hold at the top of motion and then lower back to the ground. This is one rep.

Cable Fly (Chest)

This is a good isolate move to use on your chest day as one of your variations. I like doing this very slowly. In the eccentric (downward) portion of the move, I can really feel the work that's being done. In my opinion, using cables works best, since it keeps the tension in your pecs. Using the cable crossover, grasp a pulley in each hand and bend over slightly with a straight back. Pull inward, keeping your elbows bent slightly. Return to the starting position. This is one rep.

Cable Row (Mid- to Upper Back)

A great interchangeable workout for your back routine! This helps build a substantial back and is also a good pull move to keep your upper body in balance as you do moves such as push-ups and bench presses. Using a cable rowing machine, place your feet on the platform in front of you, and bend your knees slightly. Using the V-bar, pull inward toward your lower chest. Your chest should be pushed out slightly and your back should be arched. Hold this position for a few seconds and then return to starting position. This is one rep.

Calf Raise (Legs and Calves)

This move focuses solely on one part of your leg, the calves. Either sit with weights resting on your thighs or stand holding the weights at your side or resting on your shoulders like a squat. Working from the balls of your feet, move up and down, focusing on calf flexion. As you do this exercise, imagine balancing on a step, and you'll get a better range of motion for the muscle, thus improving strength and look.

Chin-Up (Back and Biceps)

One of my top moves. I usually do this exercise toward the middle of the workout because it hits a lot of muscles. Regular pull-ups are best (using an overhand grip with palms facing away from you), but doing this afterward really stretches the lats and works the biceps. Work on a pull-up bar or anything you can hang from; use a reverse grip (palms facing toward you); and lift your chin up to the bar. Then let your body come all the way down (arms straight) and pull yourself back up.

Close Grip Bench Press (Triceps)

This is my favorite move for growing triceps. Always the first on tri-day! This is very similar to a bench press. Set up just as you would if you were doing a bench press, but keep your grip on the bar at shoulder width or just a little narrower than shoulder width. Then, keeping the elbows in, push the bar up, concentrating on the flexion of your tris. This will give you the mass in your arms you've been seeking!

Crossover Rear Lateral Raise (Shoulders and Upper Back)

Great move if you want a little more definition in your upper back. Simply find a cable station, attach a D-handle to the bottom of each side, then grab the left handle with your right hand and the right handle with your left. Standing in the middle of the cable station, bend over to about 45 degrees at the waist, be sure to lock that back in place, and bring your arms from a hanging position to straight out to your sides while focusing on your midback.

Deadlift (Legs, Core, Grip, and Upper Back)

Next to squats, this is without a doubt the best move out there. Form is incredibly important for this move, so I would highly recommend watching the video on the Ryan Ferguson Fitness channel on YouTube before performing. For safety reasons, I almost always go light on this move. Mostly because it'll build the muscle necessary to develop a strong yet slim core while also significantly reducing one's chances for injury. In my experience, and that of those whom I've worked with, it's helped build the muscle desired, while also strengthening and protecting the lower back, and I haven't had nearly as many injuries to my back since religiously incorporating this move into my routine. Plus, they work a ton of muscles all at once! Basically, you grab a barbell from the floor with a grip wider than shoulder width. Be sure to keep your feet straight, knees bent, and, most important, lock that back into place with your shoulders up. It may feel a little awkward with your butt sticking out at the bottom of this move, but that's just part of it. Don't sweat it! Begin with the bar on the floor and by activating your legs and hips, pull the barbell up to your waist. Do not round your back while lifting and remember that your arms are just there to pull the weight, not lift it.

Decline Push-Up (Chest, Shoulders, Core, and Triceps)

This move is identical to a regular push-up, except you will place your feet above floor level: a chair or a bench should work just fine. Remember, both hands on the floor, shoulder width apart, elbows in; stiffen your core with your butt lifted just a touch and then push yourself off of the floor, pause, then slowly lower back down. This can be done fast to mimic an explosive move. These are just a little more difficult than regular push-ups, since the weight distribution is centered above where you're pushing—a great progression in your calisthenics routine!

Diamond Push-Up (Chest and Triceps)

These are great for calisthenic workouts as well as at the end of a rigorous weight-exercise chest day. I enjoy incorporating these into my workouts because they seem to hit my inner pecs better than anything else I've tried, while also focusing on the triceps. Simply get into push-up position and bring your hands just inside of shoulder width. Once there, with palms flat on the ground, make a diamond shape with your hands by touching thumb to thumb and index finger to index finger. Proceed as you would with a regular push-up, but focus your energy on the inner chest and triceps. You'll feel the burn for sure!

Dip (Chest and Triceps)

I love dips. They are an awesome body-weight calisthenic movement that give you some serious triceps while also working your chest. Highly recommended. There are various ways to do dips but I would recommend sticking to a dip bar as the safest way. Simply grab the handles, lean your body a little forward and lower your body till your arms are at about a 90-degree angle. More and you run the risk of injuring your shoulders (advice I wish I knew earlier). Once down, simply push your body back till you're just about to lock out the arms. Pause and repeat.

Dumbbell Step-Up (Legs, Glutes, Core, and Forearms)

Great move for balance, while also working multiple areas of your body. Although this targets your legs primarily, it recruits many other muscles to work in unison to keep your body properly aligned. Find a box about a foot to a foot and a half off of the floor. Working with a dumbbell in each hand, simply step one foot onto the box and then the other. Step back down and repeat with your other foot first. That's one rep.

Explosive Push-Up (Chest, Triceps, and Core)

Good for working your fast-twitch muscles for speed. This move can be done one of two ways: one where you leave the ground and the other where you don't. I generally don't explode off of the ground because it hurts my shoulders and is tough on the joints. If you are like me, just do a regular push-up as quickly as possible, while still using good form, and you'll still get the benefits of an explosive movement. If you can do this move, just do a regular push-up but fast enough to leave the ground at the top of the move. Land back in the same place as you started and continue. That's it!

Front Raise (Shoulder/Front Delts)

This is a great move for improving the front of your shoulders. Not a move you should use all the time, though, because this muscle gets a lot of work from shoulder presses and bench presses, so it's easy to overdo. Simply grab a cable or dumbbell with your arm at your side, then, with your palm down, lift it up while keeping your arm straight until it is parallel to the floor, pause, and slowly bring it back down.

Hammer Curl (Biceps and Forearms)

This move will make your arms stand out for sure. I love it because I get a great pump in my arms while also working on those pesky forearms. Start by attaching the ropes you find at your cable station to one of the bottom pulleys. Then grab a side in each hand and brace your body with a slight arch in your back. Pull your shoulder blades in and lock your arms at your side. Moving at the elbow, pull the weight up to your chest, hold, and slowly bring it back down. That's one rep.

Handstand Push-Up (Shoulders, Traps, Arms, and Core)

Great upper-body move and the best there is when it comes to calisthenics. This move will build some serious strength and help add mass to your shoulder area in no time flat! Find a wall and get into a handstand position with your hands about three to six inches away from the wall and with your feet touching. Slowly lower yourself down until your head nearly touches the ground and explode back up to the top of the move. If you cannot do these yet, that's okay, just work on getting into handstand position and hold it every now and then till you find your balance. Also, use shoulder presses to help build up strength.

Hanging Leg Raise (Core, Grip, and Lower Abs)

This move is great for hitting those hard-to-reach lower abs. It is a difficult move to perform at first, so if you should find yourself having difficulty, don't get discouraged, start with lying leg raises. Grab a pull-up bar and let yourself hang from it. Then bring your knees up to your chest, being sure to rotate your hips upward, pause, and bring your legs back down to the start position. To make it more challenging, keep your legs straight instead of bending them. Also, as in other moves, do not swing or use momentum. This is unsafe for your lower back and will ultimately diminish your gains.

Inverted Row (Back, Lats, Core, and Arms)

This is one of my top moves for both calisthenics and general strength. An inverted row may look funky but once you try it you'll be hooked. They feel good! All you need is a bar and the floor. Smith machines are good for this because of their stability. Just place the bar at about midthigh height. Grab the bar with both hands so that you're hanging from it with feet out and your chest almost directly below it. Then, pull your chest up to the bar while contracting your shoulder blades; pause, and slowly bring yourself back down to the starting position.

Lateral Pull-Down (Back, Lats, and Arms)

I use this move every so often to train myself in proper technique. Although I like pull-ups more, you can change the weight with these and go light so that focusing on the movement becomes easier. Be sure to pull into your shoulder blades when doing these, just like pull-ups, and try not to use your arms. Think of them as hooks that simply move the weight your back is pulling. Also, keep a slight arch in your back when doing this move and pull the bar down to your collarbone. Go nice and slow and use this as practice for your pull-ups.

Leg Curl (Hamstrings)

Great isolation move for those all-important hamstrings. I generally pair this with leg extensions or do them by themselves on deadlift day. Either way is fine since there is really no right or wrong time to do them. This is a machine move, so it is pretty easy and self-explanatory once your find the equipment. I like the ones where you lie down on your stomach with your legs hanging off the pad from just above your knees down, and with your calves against the weighted pad. Once there, bend at the knees, curl your feet to your butt, pause, and bring it back down.

Leg Extension (Quadriceps)

This is an isolation move that is good for developing the look of your quads. One note of caution: This move can be bad for your knees if you have existing problems or attempt to go too heavy. Be realistic, however, and I believe you'll be okay. I pretty much always go light and do a lot of reps on this. Note: if you want big quads, do front squats. This move is very easy and the machine will guide you through it, but you essentially sit down as you normally would, place your shins against a pad connected to weight, and bring your legs up so that they're parallel to the floor. Easy stuff!

Long Jump (Legs)

I love this calisthenic move! It is an explosive, fast-paced movement that can be done any-where and will improve not only your strength but your speed, too. Just stand with your feet shoulder width apart, quickly crouch into jumping position, and with both feet explode forward as far as you can go. Once you land, regroup and jump again. Great explosive move. Be sure to warm up properly before performing this type of explosive movement.

Lunge and Weighted Lunge (Legs, Grip, and Core)

On leg day, it's great to do weighted lunges after squats. This exercise really works each leg individually and pushes your legs that extra mile. Grab a dumbbell in each hand; for more difficulty, work with the barbells over your head. Simply lunge one foot forward, bring the other knee almost to the ground, and push back up with the forward leg. Switch legs and you've got one rep. The routine is the same for regular lunges, but you don't use the weights.

Great calisthenics move to do anywhere! Note: you can do a full workout for each side if you wish, but I like switching it up and alternating between legs.

Lying Leg Raise (Core, Lower Abs)

Here's an easy variation on hanging leg raises. Lie on the ground, brace your body, and, keeping your legs straight, lift them and your hips up toward the ceiling. Pause at the top and slowly bring your legs back down, concentrating on the stretch in your lower abs.

Pistol Squat (Legs)

Great leg exercise to test balance and strength. Simply do a squat but balance on one foot as you extend the other foot in front.

Plank (Core)

This is one of the greatest things I've ever done for my abs. Although this works the whole core, it is a move that really made my abs stand out, and it seemed to destroy the fat that cardio alone couldn't get rid of. Get into plank position and brace your whole body. Then put your forearms on the ground instead of your hands, and hold for as long as possible. That's it. Sounds easy, I know, but I can assure you that you'll be thinking differently afterward.

Pull-Up and Weighted Pull-Up (Back and Arms)

The king of the back exercises. This will build muscle and mass with each rep; it's that great an exercise! Grab a pull-up bar a little more than shoulder width apart. Then pull your chest up to the bar by pulling your shoulder blades together; pause, then lower yourself back down. If you'd like a little extra muscle, just find a belt you can strap a weight to and go to town! If you can do this exercise weighted, I highly recommend it—it's amazing!

Push-Up, Simple Variation (Chest, Core, and Tris)

I do these daily. They are great for overall upper-body development! There is also a variation for those not yet ready for the regular version. To do these, get into regular push-up position, but use your knees as a pivot point instead of your toes. Great for beginners.

Regular Crunch (Abs)

Lie on the ground with your feet flat on the floor and your knees up. Then, lift your upper back off the floor and toward your knees. Pause for a moment and slowly bring it back down until your shoulder blades nearly touch the ground. Repeat.

Reverse Curl (Biceps and Forearms)

Great as a way to finish off your arm routine. First attach a straight bar to the bottom of a cable station. Grab the bar with a reverse grip, palms facing away from you. Then curl the bar up to your chest as you would a typical curl. That's it!

Shoulder Press (Shoulders, Traps, and Triceps)

In my opinion, this is the single best weighted move to build up the shoulders. (Handstand push-ups, a great move, using nothing but your own body's weight, may be my favorite.) All you need to do is grab either a barbell or a dumbbell in each hand and either sitting or, as I prefer, standing, take the weight from about the height of your nose to above the back portion of your head. While doing this move, it is important to keep your back slightly arched and locked into position.

Shrug (Traps)

Grab a Smith machine bar or some dumbbells and let them hang with your arms straight. Then pull your shoulders upward and back toward the rear area of your ears. It's just that easy. Be sure to have a solid stance with a slight curve in your back.

Side Crunch (Obliques)

Just like a regular crunch but done with a twist! Instead of having your legs out in front of your body, lay them to the side while keeping your shoulders in the same place. Then, crunch up and back toward your feet a little. Easy as that!

Side Raise (Shoulder/Front and Side Delts)

Similar to front raises, except now you're lifting the weight to the side of your body instead of in front of you. It's a great move, but it can overwork your frontal delts, so it's good to do this exercise sparingly as part of your shoulder routine. Grab a dumbbell or a cable, palms facing downward, and keeping your arm straight, lift it to your side, pause, and slowly bring it back down.

Single Arm Press-Down (Triceps)

Attach a D-handle to the top of a cable station. Then, grab either overhand or underhand and go from a 90-degree angle with your biceps at your side to your arm being straight, which would cause you to either push or pull the weight down. I switch it up because the different positions hit different areas of the triceps head. Something worth doing for proportion and balance.

Skull Crusher (Triceps)

Lie on a bench and grab a barbell with an overhand grip. Then bring the weight from behind your head to just above it. Slowly lower back down to behind your head and repeat.

Sled Push (Legs, Core, and Arms)

Great move for improving leg strength and power. You must work with a workout sled to perform this move. Grab the sled by the handles and, keeping a slight arch in your back, feet shoulder width apart, and slightly crouched, push the sled forward as fast as possible over a predetermined distance.

Squat (Legs, Lower Back, and Core)

This is the king of all workout moves. Studies show that this compound move works approximately 250 individual muscles. That's 250 muscles in one move! Although this is such a great move, you must also be careful when performing it. If you keep your feet forward, a slight arch in your back, and pay attention to your form, you should be just fine. I do these weekly and feel great. Watch the video for pointers on how to perform this move better.

Tri Push-Down (Triceps)

Much like the single arm press-down, tri push-downs are good to do late in your arm day or triceps workout. Either attach a rope or a straight bar to the top of a cable station, then with an overhand grip for the bar or a neutral grip for the rope, grab with your biceps at your sides and your arms at a 90-degree angle. Proceed by exerting downward force and straightening your arms out, keeping them at your sides. Pause for a moment just before you lock the arms out and slowly return to the starting position.

Wrist Curls and Extensions (Forearms)

These two moves go hand in hand and will help you develop amazing forearms. I do them at the end of every arm day, and it has paid huge dividends—especially for the short amount of time invested. Curls work the meatier bottom or back portion of your forearm while the oft overlooked extensions work the top portion. Connect a straight bar to the bottom of a cable station and lift up to your waist with your arms hanging. For extensions, pull the back of your hand toward your forearm and flex. For curls, stand the same way with the bar behind you and pull your palms up toward your forearms. Simple as that. Try doing a lot of reps and you'll feel exactly how amazing this move really is!

Acknowledgments

A special thanks to Steve Frazier Photography for several photos included in this book.

To Roger Pelegrinelli at Savannah Media for the author photographs.

To my brilliant agent, Amy Hughes, for helping me grow my writing career with her exceptional insight.

Also to my editor, Mitch Horowitz at Penguin, for helping make this book even better than I initially thought possible.

Index

Page numbers in *italics* refer to photos.

About the Author

RYAN FERGUSON spent 10 years in prison for a crime he did not commit. Today, Ryan advocates for wrongly accused people and shares the fitness program that kept him alive and healthy. He has recently appeared on *Dateline*, *Nightline*, *CBS This Morning*, *Today*, *48 Hours*, *Good Morning America*, *Katie*, *Anderson Cooper 360°*, and CNN's *New Day*. A native of Missouri, he currently lives on the Florida gulf coast and travels widely. Visit him at facebook.com/freedryanferguson and follow him on Twitter @lifeafterten and Instagram @lifeafterten.

FOR MORE INFORMATION ON RYAN'S CASE, HEALTH, AND FITNESS, PLEASE VISIT:
RyanFergusonFitness.com

TO BOOK FOR SPEAKING EVENTS:
bookings@lifeafter10.com

SOCIAL MEDIA:
facebook.com/FreedRyanFerguson
facebook.com/RyanFergusonFitness
youtube.com/RyanFergusonFitness
Twitter: @LifeAfterTen
Instagram: @LifeAfterTen

31901056102710